Instructions

LET AUGMENTED REALITY CHANGE HOW YOU READ A BOOK

With your smartphone, iPad or tablet you can use the **Hasmark AR** app to invoke the augmented reality experience to literally read outside the book.

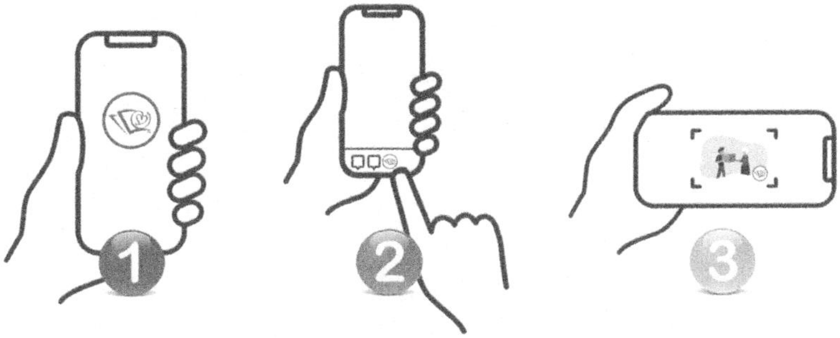

1. Download the **Hasmark app** from the **Apple App Store** or **Google Play**
2. Open and select the (vue) option
3. Point your lens at the full image with the and enjoy the augmented reality experience.

Go ahead and try it right now with the Hasmark Publishing International logo.

The Highest Frequencies of Love

The Highest Frequencies of Love

Unconventional Solutions for Parents of Children on the Autism Spectrum

Donna Laitinen

Hasmark
PUBLISHING
INTERNATIONAL

Hasmark Publishing
www.hasmarkpublishing.com

First Edition

Disclaimer

This book is designed to provide information and motivation to our readers. It is sold with the understanding that the publisher is not engaged to render any type of psychological, legal, or any other kind of professional advice. The content of each article is the sole expression and opinion of its author, and not necessarily that of the publisher. No warranties or guarantees are expressed or implied by the publisher's choice to include any of the content in this volume. Neither the publisher nor the individual author(s) shall be liable for any physical, psychological, emotional, financial, or commercial damages, including, but not limited to, special, incidental, consequential or other damages. Our views and rights are the same: You are responsible for your own choices, actions, and results.

Permission should be addressed in writing to Arthur David Krehbiel at adkrehbiel36@gmail.com

Editor: Jamie Geidel
Cover Design: Anne Karklins | anne@hasmarkpublishing.com
Interior Layout: Amit Dey | amit@hasmarkpublishing.com

ISBN 13: 978-1-77482-115-2
ISBN 10: 177482115X

Hasmark PUBLISHING INTERNATIONAL

"In her new book *The Highest Frequencies of Love*, Donna challenges readers to expand their awareness. Donna provides the tools, not just for parents with children on the autism spectrum, but for anyone who picks up this book looking to live a more intentional life."

—Peggy McColl,
New York Times Bestselling Author, www.PeggyMcColl.com

"First-time author Donna Laitinen, in her book *The Highest Frequency of Love,* teaches us about the, unique and beautiful gifts a child on the autism spectrum, brings to the lives of their caregivers. Children on the spectrum are hard-wired for authenticity, which Donna explains, is the highest frequency of love.

When we let these uniquely perfect children be our guides, we can see and appreciate their world as they need us to see it. We are then free to surrender our negative thoughts and feelings about our relationship with them and ourselves. Donna leads the reader step by step on a journey of becoming our higher and better selves - a journey to rewiring our brains for authenticity and our expression of the highest frequency of love.

This book is a practical and empowering guide for not only parents of children on the autism spectrum but for anyone who wants to understand the powerful principles of how to be their best selves."

—Dr. Joanette,
Founder of Emotional Social Parenting™,
with a neuroscience perspective. International best-selling
author of the *Giggles in my Heart* children's books
series about big emotions and feelings.

"In *The Highest Frequencies of Love,* I consistently found myself nodding along. As an expert and researcher of Posttraumatic Growth, it was a joy to experience this. Donna beautifully captures the benefits and gifts that having a child with Autism brings and shares how growth is possible for parents of these children.

I look forward to sharing this read with my clients and friends."

—Dr. Victoria Grinman,
Founder of Growing Kind Minds LLC
and Permission Slip Parenting

"Donna Laitinen's book *The Highest Frequencies of Love,* although intended for parents and caretakers of those on the Autism Spectrum, has really great tips and tactics for all of us to use in our lives to gain freedom and power. I highly recommend it."

—Scott Feld,
Partner, Author, Speaker
MindZenMotion.com

"Donna Laitinen is such a great advocate and leader in the wellness industry. I highly recommend this book."

—Robert Raymond,
CEO of Achieve Wellness Pro

"Donna's book is more than just a guide for parents with children on the autism spectrum. It is an essential tool that will allow you to tap into your authentic self to become more aware and present in your own life."

—Judy O'Beirn,
President of Hasmark Publishing International

Dedication

I dedicate this book to my dad, Edward Udas, who transitioned to the spiritual world on January 13, 2022.

Dad, you will always be the wind beneath my wings.

I feel your unconditional love wrapped around me, offering me comfort and guidance, with an invitation to dream big and grow into those dreams.

Connectivity with you has been essential in the creation of this book.

Thank you for telling me to follow my dreams and that dreamers are the innovators of the world!

Table of Contents

Prologue

October 28, 2020. That date will forever be etched in my mind. It is the date my life would change forever. It is the date that my calling, my life's true purpose, would reveal itself and simultaneously reveal my future path.

It was in the evening—the sky somewhere between the purple and pink shades of dusk and the blackness of night. I was driving home when a thought as powerful as a lightning bolt pierced my mind. It may have been dark outside, but the message was clear as a crisp, blue sky—*You are writing a book*. It was so sudden and so clear that I actually turned my head to see if someone was in the car speaking to me.

But I was alone. And I was confused. What would I write a book about? Then, as if in answer, another exceedingly powerful thought appeared—*It will help parents of children on the autism spectrum*.

For a moment, I thought it was incredibly random, but I knew better than that. "Random thoughts" are a myth; they always exist for a reason. And this reason was to provide the fuel to ignite my heart's desire—a desire that before that moment I did not even realize existed.

The adrenaline began pumping as my future path unfolded like the road in front of me. Like a one-way street, there was simply no turning back. These powerful, compelling thoughts immediately prompted decisive action. Within seconds, I called a dear friend. Her 18-year-old son, Jack, is autistic.

I explained what had just happened to me and asked for her help and for Jack's. Without hesitation, and with blind faith, she said yes—as if she had been expecting my call and question. I took a long, deep breath I didn't realize I had been holding.

During the process, the three of us (and many others along the way) trusted each other, surrendered to the path for which we were chosen, and allowed the magnificence to unfold. There was no doubt in my mind that a higher power was co-creating with us.

This book is the result of that co-creation.

This book is what happens when thoughts, energy, and action are aligned in a way to make pure magic.

Introduction

I am a firm believer in setting intentions (and I sincerely hope you are too). As such, I would like to set mine now. My intention in writing this book is to help parents of children on the autism spectrum (no matter where in the world you live) embrace the practices set forth herein so you can be the most brilliant, best version of yourself as you parent. By starting with you, you'll see that once you recondition your mind, you give permission for your child to do the same. My intention is to help bring about balance and harmony with a rekindled spirit, infusing a positive connection in the family home. As you become more balanced and in alignment in your own life, you will see the ripple effect from there. Remember—your best self is best for everyone, especially your child.

This book is intended to help parents of children with autism move obstacles out of their way. This is about truly understanding the power of the mind and implementing positive change for the long term. What makes it "unconventional" or different from other books out there is that it is more about you than your child. It's about tapping into your own internal powers and programming your mind to recognize that you are your own superhero . . . and theirs.

Throughout this book, you will discover practices that you already have the power to reach. But now, you will use your emotional intelligence to help get you there. You will examine your ability to use and manage your own emotions in positive ways to relieve stress, communicate effectively, empathize with others, overcome challenges, and defuse conflict. These practices will serve as your life raft during those times when you feel as if you are drowning.

My true heart's desire is to have you become a master of your mind, your emotions, and the practices set forth in this book through your intentions. Intention setting is one of the most powerful transformative components of healing modalities. It is what creates the flow of energy to allow your true purpose to take root and grow. Intentions are the driving force of love you wish to see in the world. Make no mistake, *you* are the solution to your inner turmoil. As your awareness, energy, and behavior begin to exude confidence and optimism, these positive attributes will affect your child in positive ways. They will begin to bridge your connection with your child's authenticity as you celebrate the natural gifts they bring to the world.

Evoking change in meaningful ways like this is my passion—my heart's desire.

The tendencies and talents of children with autism are expressed in certain unique and beautiful ways. Children on the autism spectrum don't change their personalities depending on the person they are with or the situation in which they find themselves. They don't intentionally hide their insecurities or apologize for who they are. They represent the highest frequency of love.

While their potential and influence are often overlooked in their significant contribution to the greatness in our world, they shouldn't be. What they have to offer the world truly matters—and that is pure love. My perception has shifted since engaging with Jack and so many others on this journey. They are gifts to us, and our teachers too. They teach us to be more patient, more tolerant, and more accepting of uniqueness. They teach us how to be authentic and to be our true selves. They teach us that we are all connected, and we all have great purpose.

Shouldn't we listen more to what they are telling us?

Shouldn't we pay more attention to these messages?

By following the practices in this book and our own hearts, we will clear our minds so that we can hear and see our children better.

To help guide us along this extraordinary journey, I have carefully organized each chapter to capture the true heart of the matter. You will find each chapter organized in the following way:

Positive Affirmation

All that we do starts with our intention. Repeating a positive phrase or statement as a way to challenge negative, unhelpful thoughts is an important part of setting that intention.

Sharing in the Extraordinary Journey

Life is always a journey, and each of us has a story to tell. In this section, the parents, therapists, doctors, and teachers who have contributed to this book will share a firsthand account of one of their own stories. In this way, we will connect to them and their circumstances on a more personal level.

I Grow My Wisdom

Increasing our knowledge and increasing our abilities is what we all want, right? This section gives you the building blocks to create a foundation of excellent and effective parenting. What can we learn from the story told? What are the key pieces we should take from it and why?

I Ask My True Self

Honesty and authenticity come from within. In this section, we will dig a little deeper to understand what we need to do to make changes.

Aligning Thoughts with Actions

To be the truly authentic parents our children need us to be, we need to be aware of our energy so that we can align our thoughts with our actions. This section will give you specific action items and steps to further cement your intention and make real change.

Reflections

A space that is all your own. Use it to answer *I Ask My True Self* questions and any other thoughts or reflections you had while reading that chapter.

Are you ready to make a change for the better? Are you ready to provide yourself with the support you need?

Let's begin . . .

Chapter 1

My Magnificent Mind

Releasing the Power Within

Positive Affirmation

Today I am the master of my magnificent mind and the powerhouse it is.

Sharing in the Extraordinary Journey

~ Heidi Rome, Mom and Author of You Just Have to Love Me: Drawing Strength from the Unseen

On a late winter, sunny morning in the most ordinary of places, my autistic nonverbal son gave me an unexpected glimpse of the miracles hidden in plain sight. My heart was heavy when I went into Ethan's school that day to work with him on his Spelling-to-Communicate technique, knowing that he would soon be leaving to attend a residential out-of-state placement for children with severe autism who require 24/7 high level support. In this session, about a month before he was to leave, I asked Ethan what his thoughts were about God. The subsequent conversation in which Ethan describes his experience of autism as a spiritual journey, blew me away. So much so that I later went on to write a book about it.

In response to my question, asking what we should do to help him on this tough autism journey, he typed, "You just have to love me and that is your job. The rest is my job to do." Do you hear Ethan, my fellow overwhelmed and frightened autism parents? It is not your job to fix your "broken" child. It is not your job to change another human being or make them look 'normal' like everyone else.

It is your job to love and accept them unconditionally for the complete, perfect human beings they are, each soul made in God's image. Accepting is not the same as giving up. Our job to love means to meet the other's needs, no matter what, no matter when. To be there for our child in his hardest time. To protect, educate, support, guide, and help them discover and become their own best self . . . all falls under love. This does not mean 'giving up' on them; it means accepting that which we cannot change.

I also believe that the most important step to loving your child is loving yourself first. Model what self-love and self-care look like for your child who is looking to you to be his guide. How are you treating yourself? How are you living your own life? Our sensitive kids feel our energy, our emotions—don't even try to lie to them. Be authentic, honor your own feelings—and they will witness your actions and follow suit themselves. Turn off the self-critic, turn on the self-cheerleader, and also empower your empathetic kids to do the same .

I Grow My Wisdom

Our minds have an extraordinary amount of power, and that power can be unleashed at any time. But most people don't understand how. Let's start with some basics—the conscious mind versus the subconscious mind.

Conscious Mind

The conscious mind has the ability to accept or reject any thoughts or ideas. Yes! You can control exactly what goes into your conscious mind. When you are aware of this, it is truly a game changer. Life gets simpler when you understand how to release negative thoughts and ideas from yourself, others, and circumstances, just like Heidi did.

The problem is that too often, people are on autopilot, allowing whatever is on the radio, television, or social media into their minds. They also allow other people's thoughts, ideas, beliefs, and opinions in. When these thoughts and ideas are negative or disturbing (as they often are), the body (physically) and the mind (mentally) mirror them, reflecting in your energy or vibrational output. Your actions and behaviors are a direct result of these "unwanted feelings," and they usually lead to a negative outcome.

When you encounter a negative or unwanted thought, it creates low feelings and energy output. It could be about yourself, maybe a medical condition, taking something personal that someone said, or reflecting on something you said or did that you regret. You could be worried about someone else in your life. Dwelling on it creates more unwanted feelings, and you might actually end up visualizing things to worry about—things that haven't even happened. These are illusions you create in your own mind.

When you stay in that space, recycling these negative outcomes over and over, you ignite feelings of worry, doubt, and fear, which often propel you into a state of anxiety. Before you even know it, your fear escalates, consuming you and causing you to go even deeper, putting your well-being at risk, wreaking havoc on your nervous system, and setting off physical discomfort or pain (headaches, stomachaches, loss of appetite, troubled sleep, restless muscles, exhaustion, mood swings, unproductiveness, and feeling stuck). If you stay in this pattern of worry, also known as a fight-or-flight response, depression sets in and creates a higher risk for other diseases. Negative thoughts that lead to stress affect all your major organs.

A similar process in the opposite direction holds true if you get out of autopilot and choose to focus on positive thoughts, ideas, and words. When you think positive thoughts, you create better feelings, your body generates positive energy and vibrational output, and your response is more positively driven, resulting in a more favorable result. Yes, the concept truly is that simple . . . on the surface. But it takes daily work to reprogram the mind from our automatic ways of thinking. Doing so takes awareness, desire, and committed practice. This is a habit you can begin to change today.

You have free will in the conscious mind. No person or circumstance can cause you to think about things that you do not choose to think about. When you increase your awareness, you have more control of your thoughts and invite peace of mind, clarity, and order to replace anxiety, worry, and fear. It is all up to you! Each thought you allow in creates a new feeling within you. And each feeling projects either a reaction or a response, which dictates your behavior and is directly related to the results you see. Simply, you are the ruler of your own mind, and as you develop this practice (and it is a practice), you will be able to not only catch, but to stop, the negative and worrisome thoughts before they fester and take control.

Subconscious Mind

This is where you can become whoever you want to become! The subconscious mind must accept whatever you put into it, as it has no ability to reject. That's right—any thought or idea must be accepted. When you continuously repeat or impress thoughts and words upon the subconscious mind, these ideas become fixed in your personality. You can condition your mind to your goals, your wants, and the behaviors you want to change. On the other hand, if you continually impress upon the subconscious your fears and worries and focus on what is wrong with you, you will feel more of *those* emotions. Remember—where your attention goes, your energy flows.

Now, as you direct positive thoughts to impress upon the subconscious mind, you invite more happiness and peace in. Autosuggestion is an effective tool used to deliberately reprogram the mind to improve your self-image, confidence, and self-esteem (and we will talk more about it in a later chapter). You are retraining the mind to think in a certain way. As you learn the process, adding feeling and visualization brings more energy, and this can serve to inspire ideas, choices, and events to move you toward your intention or goal.

When you learn the power of autosuggestion and positive affirmations to create your desired results within your subconscious, you can:

- Release fears
- Change habits
- Achieve goals

Talk about powerful transformations!

I Ask My True Self

- *What is my mind chattering about today?*
- *How does it make me feel—emotionally and physically?*
- *What thoughts/ideas do I want to stop from entering my mind?*
- *What thoughts/ideas do I want to welcome into my mind?*

Aligning Thoughts with Actions

- Write ten words that describe who you are.
- Write ten things you do very well.
- Write ten things you want to improve upon.
- Write ten things you want to let go of.

Reflections of the Mind . . .

Our greatest weapon against stress is our ability to choose one thought over another.

~ William James

Reflections of the Mind . . .

You become what you think about.

~ Earl Nightingale

Chapter 2

It Starts with You

Building Strength through Self-Discovery

Positive Affirmation

I have the ability to control my thoughts, energy, and actions.

Sharing in the Extraordinary Journey

~ Nicole Dauz, Mom and Founder of SelfCare4Caregivers

Self-awareness is so important for us autism parents, as it reminds us that we are separate from our children. I know it sounds obvious, but at the beginning of my caregiver journey, I was only wrapped up in my daughter's challenges and my own denial and was completely overwhelmed with what was happening all around me. Because I was in survival mode, all my attention was focused on keeping the household running, showing up at work as the 'same' employee, and telling myself that everything was good.

I was completely unaware that I was unaware.

That's the exact opposite of self-awareness, and it robbed me from accepting the situation at the beginning. As such, I was stuck in survival mode for many years to come. Now, I can't help but wonder, is this why my non-verbal daughter screamed so much? Did she feel the disconnect of my energy? Was the unawareness, unacceptance, and denial I felt a result of the inability to show up as the mother whom she needed at the time?

Things shifted for me with an incident that happened with my autistic son. It helped move me toward the inner work of self-awareness. As I entered the world of self-development, personal growth, and seeing things through another lens, I learned that just because someone says something doesn't mean it is true. This realization was at the same time that I learned that people are always projecting their thoughts and their own wants on others. I finally woke up to the fact that someone else's truth doesn't have to be my truth. I knew I had to start exploring what my truth actually was.

Then, I asked the question, "How do I feel about all of the things in my life?" My response to that question was freeing, as I started to remove the incredibly heavy weight of what others thought off my shoulders. This is when my entire life pivoted. I started along the path of following my own truth and uncovering that I was the only person responsible for my happiness.

~ Dr. Elizabeth Joy Shaffer, Mom and Therapist

I remember the day when I realized that I needed to work on my self-control, after seeing the impact of my lack of it on my kids. We were driving to school one morning, and my kids were in the back seat. Like a typical day with typical brothers, one said something, which sent the other brother into a tizzy. My youngest immediately shouted at his brother in anger and frustration. The words that came out of his mouth were not appropriate. I paused, as I was getting ready to react and impose my anger and frustration about the situation. I realized the remarks my younger son just said were the same remarks I said when I was upset a few days earlier.

At this moment, I realized it was more important for me to work on my self-regulation and self-control before working on my child's. This experience prompted my healing and self-care journey. Fast forward three years, both of my boys are much calmer and able to handle strong emotions, just as I am. I "showed" them how, but it had to start with me first. If we want our children to learn self-control, we must first embrace this lesson for ourselves.

It is not always easy to have self-control as a parent when you are burning the candle at both ends. Raising children with autism takes a lot of physical and mental energy. And we only have so much energy to use in a day, so we must be mindful of where we spend it. Knowing this, I began to reflect on where my mind was most of the time. I realized how much time and mental energy I was spending thinking about injustices, while trying to get support for my children and meeting resistance from others. These moments would often send me into a rant, which I would continue to ruminate over for several days after the event.

These internal battles left me with little patience and energy for myself and my children. Life got much easier when I became more mindful of my thoughts and had more self-control over which thoughts I would let go of and which ones I would follow. I began to have more compassion toward myself and others during these difficult situations, which helped me to let go of the anger and frustration I felt toward them. Parents of children with autism are often "fighting" for their children.

Fighting took a lot of energy from me, so I began to take a more diplomatic approach to helping my children. I brought empathy, compassion, and a positive mindset to all sides of the situation instead of my armor, anger, and frustration. When I did this, I found those who worked with my child were much more willing to listen to, and support, my requests for helping my son once I changed my emotional state. Having more self-control over my emotional state was one of the best gifts I could have given my children.

~ Adam Szecowka, Dad, Spectrum Specialist, and
Global Energy Healer

Self-discipline requires practice in mastering your thoughts. You will see the most improvement when it becomes the catalyst in responding the way you want in connecting with your child, especially when dealing with meltdowns. When challenges associated with autism arise, having a conscious response can be more beneficial for all concerned. This is the difference between a reaction and a response.

It has been proven by the Heart Math Institute that a child with autism is wired differently biologically, with involuntary survival instincts. This means when the child is showing challenging behavior or having a meltdown, it is not their fault. Respond in a way that reflects this to the child, letting them know you don't blame them.

This also means that your child experiences a threat in a situation that may seem completely innocent to you. They may experience a fight, flight, or freeze response that manifests itself in a tantrum or meltdown. When we are aware and have enough self-discipline not to react to the behavior and instead, show up with compassion, we can then nurture their emotional and physical well-being.

I Grow My Wisdom

As we can see from these amazing stories, self-discovery, including awareness, control, and discipline is a crucial prerequisite to developing the skills required for mental, emotional, and physical strength. With strength comes the preparedness and resilience to better equip you for the challenges you face daily.

It begins with reflection and an active awareness of your behaviors, habits, and reactions. Pay attention to your thoughts and feelings. They are a powerful influence on your words and actions. Make the conscious decision to stay grounded with appropriate responses, rather than rash reactions. Set an intention and visualize it. Visualizing gives energy to your intention that will last throughout your day. Outward change will always begin internally in your mind and heart.

As you develop awareness and control of your thoughts and feelings, your words and actions will follow, and so will your energy. This energy affects all that is around you—most importantly, your children. They learn from your cues, even if you don't feel as if they are. You are planting seeds with your words, actions, behavior, and attitude. And those seeds will grow in your children, with you as their guide.

Self-awareness

Everything begins with self-awareness. Self-awareness is the ability to notice your thoughts and to feel how they influence your behavior. It is your personal power. With self-awareness, you can harness your inner strength and stand a little taller. As you continue to become more aware, you are building your personal power and developing your personal strength.

So many of us exist on autopilot—just trying to survive another day. But it shouldn't be like that. And our behaviors and actions directly influence others, especially our children. Your children don't understand that you aren't thinking and feeling the same as them. They also likely have trouble reading social cues. It's not that they don't care about other people's feelings. Instead, they may not notice or understand them. They have no choice . . . but we do. Self-awareness is a skill that can be developed over time. When one understands oneself better, it is easier to build positive self-esteem and recognize inner strengths. We begin operating at a different frequency. And the first ones who will benefit (after ourselves, of course) are our children.

It's simple, really. *Conscious self-awareness leads to conscious parenting*. A better understanding of yourself through connections to your thought processes and your behaviors is the goal. As you continue your journey of self-discovery, your children and all those around you will reap the benefits. When you become acutely aware of your thoughts, words, feelings, and actions, you are deciding to release the conditioning, also known as the clutter in your mind, allowing clarity and space to nurture good thoughts. Far too often, we are consumed with fear, doubt, and worry, so the good thoughts, ideas, and feelings do not stand a chance. We get in our own way and prevent feeling good. As you practice and learn to decide what enters your mind, you bring freedom to concentrate on what matters.

With awareness that you have a choice to free your mind of the fear-based thoughts, you become more energized, raising your vibration. Then, the skill of sharpening your intuition to lead the way occurs naturally. Increased awareness is the natural feeling of connectedness to your inner being—your instincts, gut feelings, and intuition.

Self-control

Realizing we have the choice to either respond or react is a monumental discovery with self-control. Without awareness, we nearly always go into a reactionary mode filled with worry, fear, and exaggeration. We think it is our job to fix everyone. We think we know better. But often others don't want us to fix them. Rather, they want someone to listen. Just listen. Do you have enough self-control to do that?

Think about being part of the solution by stepping back and inviting a safe space for this person or situation instead of reacting with elevated emotions based on what you think. People who immediately react usually do not come up with the best solution, as they are coming from a space of their own fear-based thoughts. Reactors proceed with limited information due simply to immediately going into "I have to fix" mode, and not taking the time to listen and understand the situation fully.

Instead, with self-control, decide to make a choice to respond politely and with calmness. By doing that, you are choosing to protect your energy and not get sucked in by theirs. You just took your power back. Choose not to elaborate if you don't want to have a discussion. Otherwise, this conversation could quickly bring your energy down, consuming your mind and precious time if you allow it to. Once again, you are in control of the situation. You are not judging, you are observing, and managing your emotions by responding. Mission accomplished—now practice!

Moving forward, when you feel your emotions elevate into reaction mode, stop, pause, and take a breath. Ask yourself, is this about me and my feelings? How can I support and encourage, not judge or ridicule? Now, you are responding. Maybe offer a different view of the situation in a brighter light, looking for the good that could come out of the situation. The mind is open now to finding a solution. As you choose to respond, your mind is able to process better, making room for rational, logical ideas to flow.

Today, commit to becoming the observer of yourself. Set an intention to only respond. Setting an intention creates awareness, which creates energy. This will take practice, so if you do not catch the behavior right away and you choose to react, do not beat yourself up. Honor yourself for being aware, and next time this happens, know you will try again to respond rather than react. You are changing your old habits and reconditioning your mind to become the version of you that you desire . . . and that your children need.

Self-discipline

Make no mistake, self-discipline is a true marker of self-love. Self-discipline is the ability to give yourself a command and then follow it. When you honor your "word," you honor yourself, and when you honor yourself, you love yourself. We follow commands from others all day long. We are so committed to everyone else and to not letting them down. Why can't we be that committed to not letting ourselves down?

Self-discipline can be challenging based on our paradigms. A paradigm is a mental program—subconscious conditioning that develops throughout our lives from childhood through adulthood based on our upbringing and experiences and our reactions to them. Our paradigm literally shapes our thought patterns and beliefs about everything, and it creates direct results in our behaviors. We all have them. It is our mental conditioning that is impressed on our mind from others. This occurs while we are growing up, and our parents, grandparents, and teachers impress their own beliefs onto us. There is no ill intention—it is just how life has always worked generally. However, once we recognize this, we can begin to change the mental conditioning we grew up with and reprogram our minds to align with *our own* beliefs. This results in being more disciplined.

Positive infusion is something we need daily for self-discipline. Start your day with positivity and share it with your children. Find good things to say to start your morning within your home. You can find plenty of motivational messages on the internet if you need help. Make them simple though—what will your child understand? This is a way to positively engage with your children and raise their power within. It will do wonders for your child and for you!

Empowering our children, building their confidence so they recognize they are valued and what they have to say is worthy, ignites the spark of internal motivation to be more, do more, and give more. This also allows you and your children to have more balance and peace within. This is how we build self-discipline. Our children hear us, even though we sometimes don't think they do. Release your expectations and be open to the unexpected. Know with confidence that your words are being heard, so choose them wisely.

I Ask My True Self

- *How often do I notice my thoughts and feel how they influence my behavior?*
- *How can I protect my energy from others' negativity?*
- *Do I respond or react?*
- *How can I respond more and react less?*
- *What can I do to be more disciplined in my daily activities?*

Aligning Thoughts with Actions

As with all progress, the journey of self-discovery will take time and practice.

For self-awareness:

- Add quiet time (10–15 minutes) to your morning or evening routine. Write your intentions down. What are you thinking about? How are you feeling? Writing helps provide additional awareness and energy.
- Be present in more conversations or situations each day.
- Take notice of how your energy affects your children.
- Be aware of the words you use—remember, words hold your energy and have an impact. They are your wand.
- Choose one thing you can do to work toward a goal and share it with someone who will help you be accountable for it.

For self-control, especially when interacting with your children during challenging times:

- Take a step back and truly observe the situation, not just the actions involved, but your energy with the intentions behind those actions.
- Intentionally take responsibility for your energy and your reactions.
- Try this one-minute breathing exercise to prevent reacting:
    - Inhale for five seconds, hold your breath for five seconds, and slowly exhale for five seconds.

- Ask yourself—Am I fueling the tension and making the situation worse or am I trying to calm the situation?
- Don't say a word to your child at this time. Be quiet. Think about what your face looks like. Let it show compassion. (Remember, your child is having a hard time because their energy is out of balance. Their behavior is not intentional.)
- If you must talk, use a soft, compassionate tone, using one or two words.

After repeating and perfecting the above exercise, you will start to see that you have more control than you ever did before.

Follow this powerful mindset road map to self-discipline:

- Know what you want.
- Know what you don't want.
- Declare your want, your desired change, or a new habit you want to establish.
- Commit to writing, visualizing, and taking action toward your desired change daily.
- Include daily rituals, including meditation, gratitude, prayer, yoga, and exercise.
- When faced with a situation that requires willpower, ask, "What choice will best help me get to my goal?"
- Face challenges and struggles with an eagerness to find a better way.
- Learn to love the struggle, as that is when we grow the most.
- Remember to rule your mind, or it will rule you.
- Remember that knowledge is power, and self-knowledge is self-empowerment.
- Remind yourself why you're striving for your goal in the first place.
- Never beat yourself up when you slip, as it is part of the process.

- Stop negative self-talk—it brings you to a low vibration or low energy state of mind.
- Schedule weekly check-ins with your accountability partner.

Reflections of Self-awareness and Self-control . . .

Self-awareness gives you the capacity to learn from your mistakes as well as your successes. It enables you to keep growing.

~ Lawrence Bossidy

Reflections of Self-discipline . . .

Self-discipline begins with the mastery of your thoughts. If you don't control what you think, you can't control what you do.

~ Unknown

Chapter 3

Find Your Hidden Potential

Tapping Into Your Higher Faculties

Positive Affirmation

Today all of my hidden potential will manifest itself openly and freely.

Sharing in the Extraordinary Journey

~ Nicole Dauz, Mom and Founder of SelfCare4Caregivers

If being a parent of a child with autism and a rare genetic disease has taught me anything, it's the chance to celebrate ALL victories. We must find the magic in all progress and happily throw the unattainable idea of perfection out the window!

It's learning and accepting that our child's progress isn't linear. It's staying positive during those moments of plateau (and even regression) and holding onto hope that progress will return. My family has so much fun celebrating when my daughter learns a new word at twelve years old. There's nothing like when she pronounces a known word with such clarity that a guest understands what she's saying.

I've recently taught my daughter, Summer, to say, "Summer is smart." And it brings such a smile to her face. I can feel the pride in her voice when she says it. That's progress at its best!

~ Richard Schreiber, Dad and Founder,
NYC Autism Community Group

Children, especially those with autism, may become easily disappointed or frustrated when they fail to accomplish something or when circumstances around them do not match their expectations. They may direct their frustration onto others, causing friction with people.

My sixteen-year-old daughter struggles when things do not go according to her plan. In my role as a father, I constantly convey to her this important message:

It's frustrating when things don't go our way! But if we change that one belief—that instead of things happening to us, they happen for us—when things don't quite go according to plan, we can just shrug it off, learn from it, and say "better luck next time!" Of course, luck has nothing to do with it. Now, my daughter rebounds quickly because she knows that missteps can be remedied by keeping her attitude positive and trying again until she gets it right. I'm often amazed at my daughter's resilience in these moments—a true source of pride for her father!

I Grow My Wisdom

When you expect things to go your way, there is less resistance to receive what you want. When you set this positive tone for the day, there is more ease and less worry and self-doubting energy, and you move through the day expecting things will happen the way you want them to. You bring about what you think about.

Remember, the vibration you go to sleep with is the vibration you wake with. The word vibration simply means energy. Going to bed with worry will only make you wake up with more of that same energy. The last thing you want is to wake up feeling exhausted and unmotivated. Try setting an intention the night before, declaring how you want the next day to go. And expect things to go your way. You are the only one who can set the trajectory for your day. That is the secret ingredient!

Forming a habit of setting an intention at bedtime allows for more comfort for the night's sleep, expecting the next day to go well. Again, the more you imprint the idea in your mind, the more power and energy you give to your belief in it, and the more your behavior will reflect it. Visualize this intention, as if your mind is a great movie screen showing the scene playing out in vivid detail. This is developing control of your thoughts, feelings, and behavior. Creative energy thinking is a science and a skill you can develop.

If you find yourself anxious about something coming up with your child, set an intention. Brainstorm and come up with some positive phrases. Say them out loud several times before bed and then again upon waking. You are consciously shifting your vibration. The idea is not to swing back and forth from one end of the emotional pendulum to the other, keeping you in a low vibrational space. When you do that, you set yourself up to be sucked into the hurricane. But as always, it takes practice to stay grounded and centered.

Choosing frustration instead of acceptance leads to low vibration, low self-image, and feeling disappointed in yourself. When you are learning and practicing something new, you never want to feel bad, disappointed, or frustrated. Sometimes you will catch the negative thoughts and words and sometimes you won't. Progress over perfection is truly the key here. The goal is to find yourself in a space where this happens more naturally and eventually becomes the way you speak to yourself and others. Basically, this is an entirely new love language. You are setting boundaries for your inner critic.

Tap Into Your Higher Faculties

To truly find your hidden potential, you must unlock your higher faculties. This is the task of becoming the person you want to be. There are so many things people want to do in their lives. They're motivated, but something holds them back. As we continue to think in a certain way and act in a certain way, with self-love and compassion for all, nothing will hold us back. By bringing awareness to your higher faculties, you can massively increase your potential and the odds to live a life you love.

So, what are your higher faculties? They are imagination, intuition, perception, reason, will, and memory.

Imagination: A miracle tool that allows you to find wonder in the mundane and become a vessel for creative ideas to flow.

Imagination is more powerful than knowledge.

~ Thomas Edison

Intuition: What many call your sixth sense. It is what you refer to when you say, "Something doesn't feel right." Its message is an energy frequency that is in alignment with the infinite—a spiritual prompting or personal revelation. It is easy to dismiss your "gut feeling," but you shouldn't. When you are in tune with your intuition, you are more powerful to predict outcomes and make wise choices.

If you want the truth, I'll tell you the truth: Listen to the secret sound, the real sound, which is in you.

~ Kabir

Perception: The source of your point of view and your perspective. By exercising your ability to change your perception, you can shed limiting beliefs that block you or hold you back.

When you change the way you look at things, the things you look at change.

~ Wayne Dyer

Reason: The ability to be consciously aware of the thoughts and ideas that come to your mind, and to choose to reject or accept them into your reality. This is undoubtedly one of the most treasured gifts that God, or our higher power, gave you—the ability to choose what images you hold in your mind to create your results.

You become what you think about.

~ Earl Nightingale

Will: The mental faculty that gives you the ability to focus only on one idea and exclude everything else. This is an ability required to succeed at anything and can be illustrated by any success story you can imagine. To create success, you must filter out negative thoughts, habits, and people. This mental strength can be developed through practice because what you focus on expands.

Only those that risk going too far can possibly find out how far one can go.

~ T.S. Eliot

Memory: This is a muscle that you can (and should) exercise. You can have a trained memory or an untrained one. Learn skills that use brain plasticity to improve your capacity to memorize and store information. There are even books to develop skills to remember names, places, and things.

What we don't use, we lose.

~ Jimmy Connors

Micro Wins for the Big Results

When you get discouraged or things aren't progressing as fast as you would like, remember— micro wins add up to big results! It takes time to implement new habits, new awareness, and new attitudes for the long term. It is a daily practice. It's okay if your thoughts go into that negative space or your words are less than kind. With practice, you will begin to recognize the flashpoints that start these negative spirals and have the opportunity to stop them before they happen. Know that it is okay, and that this is the process of reprogramming your mind. Embrace the grind as a challenge to choose better next time. The fact that you are aware of the negative thoughts or words is progress!

Here's a personal example. One of my goals is to stay out of the "treat" cabinet because I am trying to eat healthier. The first time I encountered the treat cabinet after I made this goal, I just opened it and took a treat anyway. Then I remembered my goal. (A micro win—I remembered). I said, "Next time, I will do better." At the second occurrence, I paused and asked myself, "Does this help me get to my goal?" I chose to open the treat cabinet, take out a treat, but then put it back. (Another micro win.) At the third occurrence, I was aware but took the treat anyway, and then noticed how that made me feel and said, "The next time I will do better." (A micro win.) For the fourth occurrence, I opened and closed the treat cabinet several times, and then chose to take a treat, but I tried to identify why I had the impulse to go there in the first place. (Another micro win.) At the fifth occurrence, I opened and closed the treat cabinet as I asked myself, "Does this help me get to my goal?" By the sixth time, I looked at the treat cabinet and chose not to open it. (A micro win.) Now, I never open the cabinet, as I have changed my behavior and broken the habit. (A big win.) It takes time. It is progress over perfection.

I also often play the WIN BIG challenge, a mental battle where I challenge myself to have ten wins in one day. For example:

- I got up this morning and smiled . . . WIN #1
- I meditated for ten minutes . . . WIN #2

- I set an intention today to have courage . . . WIN #3
- I wrote down five things I was grateful for . . . WIN #4
- I caught myself saying a negative word and turned it into a positive . . . WIN #5
- I looked at myself in the mirror and said, "I am strong; I am amazing" . . . WIN #6
- I said something nice to someone who usually annoys me . . . WIN #7
- I listened to a podcast on something I want to learn about . . . WIN #8
- I journaled my thoughts today . . . WIN #9
- I sang a song out loud and broke out in dance . . . WIN #10
- I laughed today . . . EXTRA BIG WIN

I Ask My True Self

- *What things do I beat myself up over?*
- *When do I get frustrated?*
- *How does that make me feel?*
- *How does that affect my energy?*
- *How can I change my self-talk to progress toward my goal?*
- *What do I want to happen tomorrow?*
- *Is there something that I want to go a certain way tomorrow?*

Aligning Thoughts with Actions

- Challenge yourself to have ten WINS today—count them; write them down.
- State your intention for tomorrow before you go to bed tonight.
- Expect things to go your way.
- Recognize your higher faculties. How do they serve you?

Reflections of the Potential . . .

Believe you can, and you're halfway there.

~ Theodore Roosevelt

Reflections of the Potential . . .

Intuition is your soul whispering the truth to your heart
and hoping that you hear.

~ Kate Spencer

Chapter 4

Attitude Is Everything

Habit of the Heart

Positive Affirmation

Today I am eternally grateful for all that I have.

Sharing in the Extraordinary Journey

~ Richard Schreiber, Dad

Your attitude should always begin from the perspective that life is happening *for* you, not *to* you. That is the backbone of being positive in life. It is something I impress upon my daughter every day. My daughter also grasps the concept of gratitude (although as a teenager, this is a hidden gem most of the time!).

My daughter, Katarina, once attended a weekend youth seminar where other kids her age shared about being raised in a divorced environment or facing other challenges that she takes for granted. That was very insightful for her. She was being raised surrounded by a loving family, who tells her each and every day she is loved and supported.

Katarina also has had every need taken care of by her parents consistently and with love. Because of this, she is not the least bit materialistic and is happy with what she has. Her attitude permeates with positivity in spite of her gravitation toward satire and dark humor, which she extends without malice, but rather with innocence.

~ Heidi Rome, Mom and Bestselling Author *of You Just Have to Love Me: Drawing Strength from the Unseen*

I had flown out of state to be with Ethan on his 14th birthday. His case manager had arranged an autumn-time special activity for our time together, so we took our collected fallen leaves and dried out sticks into a large gym with mats along the edges. I was sitting on a mat on one side of the huge room tracing leaves with crayons. Ethan was on a mat on the opposite side, methodically breaking sticks into tiny pieces and crumbing those into dust. At some point, he finished his task and proceeded to take off his shoes and socks and started to smell his feet.

I felt myself react and noticed the harsh thoughts flying through my head: *Oh shoot, I wish he wouldn't do that. That's so weird. He is 14. That is something a two-year-old does. What if someone sees him?* Then, I stopped myself. I said to my inner, judging self, *Heidi, so what? Feet do smell interesting. We've all smelled our feet! And that is not important. Why focus on that? You're here. You're here with your child on his birthday. This is the most wonderful day. How lucky and blessed you are. He is the most adorable guy. Look at those cheeks. He does have those squeezy cheeks. I just love him so much.*

I thought about Ethan's magnetic giggle that people hear and then smile and turn around to see who has that angel's laugh. I felt my body relax, and I smiled, and sat gazing at my beautiful boy with full throttle love. What happened, I realized later, was that I shifted out of my anger and fear of judgment, and into focusing on how much joy he brought me just from his presence. All of these thoughts were swirling in my head, though externally it all only took a short time. A few minutes went by, and Ethan was no longer paying attention to his feet. I watched as he got up and crossed the gym to me. He then sat next to me and without a sound lay his head in my lap. If time could have stood still forever, in that magical moment, all would have been well with the world. It struck me that he actually felt the attitude SHIFT in me—the transformation when I moved out of anger and into love and gratitude.

In my story, I did not suppress the anger and sadness I felt upon Ethan's behavior of smelling his feet. Those strong emotions are signals of our humanity; they were my wake-up call in that moment showing me what I was choosing to focus on. They were messages from my brilliantly designed, fabulously wise body's chemical and electrical communication system. They weren't wrong or bad; they just were. We don't get to pick and choose the feelings we want to feel or not feel; if we suppress one, we suppress all. Yet, we need them all, as they all contribute to our life experience, just as all tastes contribute to our experience of the foods we eat. When we eat, we can't say, "I choose to only taste sweet, not bitter."

We must name, feel, and own our feelings, our own truth of experience. Besides, our sensitive kids feel everything we feel anyway; no sense in denying your reactions, as they will know immediately if you are lying. If you insist on saying all is fine when you feel like a wreck, your child will know that what he hears and what he knows do not match. That is unsettling and dysregulating for our kids; they feel you do not trust them with the truth; they learn to doubt their own instincts and feel disempowered. Be genuine, love and honor yourself enough to share what's real for you in the moment, and model that authenticity that reinforces that you are both perfect as you are and very brave in your approach to life's challenges.

~ Nicole Donovan, Mother of four, Author of *A Life Suspended: A Mother and Son's Story of Autism, Extinction Bursts, and Living a Resilient Life*

Jack was diagnosed at seven years old, after being expelled from first grade due to behavioral issues. After his expulsion, we sought answers through intensive testing, and he was diagnosed with high-functioning autism. By this time, due to the stress, trauma, and years of being misunderstood, Jack's emotional and physical regulations were non-existent. We spent months with professionals implementing an individualized education program (IEP) with therapeutic support. As Jack's body and mind began to regulate, he was able to begin to heal the trauma and build his self-esteem.

One of the most powerful tools we used during this time was Jack's Success Book. We filled a binder with photos, awards, and stories of Jack's successes. Jack's therapist, Robin, was the initial creator of this project. It was part scrapbook and part therapy log, all pointing to Jack's milestones with photographs and captions with positive affirmations. Jack and I would read through his Success Book as we added to it. If he was having a tough day, it was there to remind him of all the ways he was successful. For a child with autism, to have a visual tool with a history of positive outcomes was profound.

In addition, I collected facts and articles about well-known people who were diagnosed with ASD, like Dan Aykroyd. One night we watched a clip from the film *Blues Brothers* of him singing and dancing. We viewed the movie *Ghostbusters* and saw how funny he was in his role as Ray Stantz, one of the team of scientists who battled supernatural creatures with high-tech gadgets.

We talked about famous men in business and historical figures who had been suspected of having ASD due to their quirky and brilliant natures. Jack liked hearing about how smart they were and how they were often perceived as "different" by society and peers. Jack particularly loved the story about Albert Einstein and how he forgot to put on his pants one day before leaving his house. I explained that Einstein knew he needed to wear pants before he went out, but his brain was so busy thinking about other things, he forgot. Jack could identify. Jack started to recognize he was not alone.

Each week, when Jack had his therapy appointment with Robin, they added another page to Jack's book. During these sessions, they pulled out successful threads from the past week, creating a visual list. The remarkable items ranged from earning a sticker to using positive language. My personal favorite was, "I succeed at everything!" Jack was getting into the groove by making positive choices each and every day. To see it compiled in one place was empowering for all of us!

I Grow My Wisdom

Attitude is everything! A positive attitude moves you forward. A negative attitude drags you down, sucking all of your energy and even the energy of those around you.

Attitude is a combination of your thoughts, feelings, and actions. Have you ever noticed that people with good attitudes are easier to talk to, easier to get along with, and easier to do business with? They exude confidence, optimism, and assurance. You can feel it instantly when they walk into a room. People want to be around people who have good attitudes—they are magnets because, on some level, we all want to feel like that. It is your attitude toward life which will determine life's attitude toward you, and it is your attitude toward others which will determine their attitude toward you.

The Attitude of Gratitude

When consciously in gratitude, it is impossible to be in a negative state of mind! You simply cannot be in a state of gratitude and have a negative mindset at the same time. Gratitude eradicates worry, so start today. In this moment, take a deep, long breath and be grateful for your heart beating and for the sun rising with its light and heat that are essential for life to grow. Give thanks for the raindrops from the sky to keep everything alive and vibrant. Think of the rain as a "cleansing" of the earth and find gratitude even for this new attitude toward rain. *Choose to feel the rain; don't just get wet.*

Be grateful for your heart beating. Be thankful for your legs, so you can walk and get to where you need to go—not everyone is so lucky. Do you ever think to be grateful for the air you breathe? We all take from it and there is always more, but how many times do we really consider that? Take a moment to recognize all of the abundance and limitlessness in the universe, and then recognize all the abundance and limitlessness within you!

With each pause, each moment of giving thanks, your heart opens a little more. You begin to feel and listen more from your heart and less from mind chatter or your inner critic. It is magical when you experience the shift in your energy through the power of gratitude. It simply and quietly calms the internal tornado that swirls within you.

Love and kindness emanate from your being through your actions, igniting the inner spark of internal motivation. Transformation of your being brings a peace and joy that is indescribable. Practicing gratitude is life's path to alignment with all the good you desire. As you create balance and harmony within yourself, you are leading others intrinsically, including your children, just by shining your beam of light and sharing your words of wisdom.

Complaining and focusing your attention on pain will only mirror and reflect negative energy. Try to keep your mind open to release the pain and think of the outcome you desire, bringing gratitude and attention to all the good you do have in your life. This habit alone can radically change your perception and well-being.

When someone says something critical of you or a situation, try some of these alternative phrases:

- Begin your response with "Thank you."
- "I will take another look at that," and move on.
- "I see your point, that is interesting," and move on.
- "I value your opinion. My thoughts are different, and that is okay."
- "I will give some thought to what you said and get back to you."

With this approach, you protect your energy by not engaging in a defensive way. You respond rather than react. Ultimately, you want to welcome criticism as a good thing, as there may be some truth in it that helps you learn something about yourself, so you can strive to do better. Forward vision thinkers thank critics, as it may be an opportunity to see more clearly. Reprogramming the mind to think a certain way takes practice. You are developing more awareness of how you want to feel, with less focus on ego.

Faith vs. Fear

I encourage you to consider how you can live so that your inner beliefs and outward actions are in alignment. It's time to consider a faith versus fear attitude. And to do this, you must believe in the invisible for both. You have the ability to consciously decide to live in faith or to live in fear. This is about having compassion and responding from a place of kindness and determination to heal. Faith is born of gratitude with an intention of thinking and acting in a certain way, as well as expecting things to go your way. A grateful mind is devoted to thinking of the best outcome for all, which positively infuses faith.

And cultivating the habit of being grateful for every good thing that comes to you increases that faith.

Faith: Always looking for the good in any situation. Believing that no matter how bad things get, knowing with certainty that something good will come out of the fire. Being able to relax with a sense of knowing that everything will be okay in the end and having the mindset to give heart and light to the situation.

Fear: Obsessing over your wounds, recycling the old "should have/could have" scenarios, and playing the blame game keeps you from moving forward. You remain stuck in this space, as you become consumed with worry, fear, doubt, confusion, frustration, anger, and uncertainty, all of which fuel the burning fire. Fear brings chaos to a higher level and invites anxiety and depression into our hearts.

Faith: You believe in natural miracles. You ask for help. You ask for guidance. You ask for people to be put in your path to help you. You ask to place events in your life to lead you on a better path. You know you are worthy of the good you desire. You know you are co-creating. You believe in a higher power.

Fear: You believe that miracles don't happen to people like you. You hold the belief that you are not worthy of a natural miracle. You fear that you are not good enough or deserving of a miracle. You don't ask for help or guidance or attempt co-creating with a higher power. You don't believe in a higher power. You look for someone or something to blame for your problems and ask questions like, "Why me? What is wrong with me?"

Faith: You embrace what you want, and you are open to the unexpected. You have the confidence that you do not need to have it all figured out to move forward, because you know that help is on the way. You recognize that all obstacles are opportunities for you to grow and walk your path and that these are the stepping-stones to something better. All your good and bad experiences have shaped you into the person that you are.

As you grow your wisdom and live more from your heart space and less from the ego, there is more of a willingness to surrender. You cultivate this awareness through daily practice, honoring your own relationship with the universe and inviting guidance. Pray for motivation to allow the power of discipline to guide your life and allow you to focus on your desired goals and pursue them with strength and conviction. Ask for kindness to emanate from your being through all your actions to let go, forgive, and forge ahead with a rekindled spirit. With practice, you will be able to answer your own questions by connecting with your inner self.

Fear: You're stuck in a tornado that is spiraling out of control in confusion, but you know this as your baseline, as your way of life, and you are comfortable in this space no matter how much chaos is there. Know that this is okay. Each of us has our own journey—our own path in our own time. When you're ready for a shift, you will know it; you will feel it. Fear of the unknown, fear of change, fear of imperfection, fear of not being smart enough, not being lovable, and being alone is what keeps you in this tornado. Stop listening to the harmful mind chatter and start listening with your heart.

I Ask My True Self

- *How is my attitude?*
- *What are ten things I am grateful for today?*
- *What was my favorite part of the day?*
- *Whom did I help today?*
- *Did I give a compliment to someone?*
- *What is one thing I want to happen tomorrow?*
- *What is my gift to share?*
- *What is my purpose?*
- *Does that make my heart glow or dim?*
- *Do my thoughts, feelings, actions, and results show up as fear or faith?*
- *Do I like the results I am getting in my life?*

Aligning Thoughts with Actions

- Think of ways you can improve your attitude in general and in certain situations. Follow these steps to building a bulletproof attitude:
  - Set the attitude for the day to be more productive in everything you do. Declare it!
  - Say, "I am bringing everything to the party—all I've got!"
  - Give more of yourself to others. Make it a habit. Each day, make someone's day better because they had an interaction with you. As you uplift others, you will uplift your own attitude. Take the mindset, "I willingly give and graciously receive."
  - Start and end each day with gratitude. This can be as simple as journaling, meditating, or silently thinking of three to five things for which you are grateful.
- Write down your answers to these questions:

  1. Do you think you have a positive attitude? Why?
  2. Would family and friends say that you have a positive attitude? Why?
  3. Would you say you flow with the current of life or against it? Why?
  4. Do you see the world we live in as a wonderful place?
  5. How do you want your child to view the world?
  6. Are your answers reflecting the results you want in your life?

Reflections of Attitude . . .

Life will bring you pain all by itself. Your responsibility is to create joy.

~ Milton Erickson

Reflections of Attitude . . .

Life is like a camera. Focus on what is important. Capture the GOOD TIMES. Develop from the negatives and if things don't work out, TAKE ANOTHER SHOT.

~ Unknown

Chapter 5

The Art of Visualization

Life's Coming Attractions

Positive Affirmation

Today I am the creator of my vision . . . and my reality.

Sharing in the Extraordinary Journey

~ Dr. Elizabeth Joy Shaffer, Mom and Therapist

Forward vision thinking is an excellent tool for us and for our kids. As parents, we often feel we need to be perfect and we must do everything on our own, or we are perceived as weak. We are often conditioned not to ask for help, and then beat ourselves up when we make mistakes. When we act this way, our kids see it, feel it, and model our behavior. We must show our kids it is okay to make mistakes. Mistakes are opportunities to learn and grow.

Sometimes our kids on the spectrum get very upset when they make mistakes because they know what they want to do, but they can't always do it that way. When my son made one little mistake in preschool, he would immediately rip up his entire paper. He hated making mistakes, so we had to show him it was okay, and that it takes practice before one can get good at something. During the practice stage, we must know that things will not look the way we always want them to, which is part of the learning process. Just as making mistakes is part of the learning process and moving forward is just as important. So, begin using these words, "Let's move forward." We can't go back and change what happened, so let's start where we are and move forward. This is such an important concept for our children. Model for your child that it is truly okay to make mistakes, then say, "This is a learning opportunity, and I will think about what just happened and how I can do it differently next time."

Forward vision thinking with self-reflection is a great tool to reflect positively and not judge. When I make a mistake, I say, "Oops, I made the wrong decision, but looking at it now, I can see that this is a better choice."

I Grow My Wisdom

You are always manifesting what you are thinking, visualizing, believing, and feeling, whether consciously or unconsciously, and so is your child. In fact, individuals with autism have an extremely strong ability to visualize, so this is a technique that should be used often with them. They are naturally very good at it.

Manifesting consciously means declaring your desires and directing your energy toward them. Simply put, manifestation is the idea that what you put out to the universe comes back to you in time through new realities. This is a process of calling in the vibration of what you ultimately want to embody and is known as the Law of Attraction, one of the universal laws. The Law of Vibration is the law that serves as the foundation of the Law of Attraction. If you are new to these universal laws, I encourage you to learn more—you have absolutely nothing to lose and an abundance to gain to ignite your internal motivation.

Allow your thoughts to reflect your desired vibration or energy output. High or low, it is up to you. Simply, if you activate sad or negative images and thoughts in your mind, you move into a negative vibration, making it almost impossible to achieve your goals. Develop the skill to kick up your vibration to higher levels so that others around you, and particularly, your children, become happy just being with you. And when you practice kindness with intention, it becomes another positive habit and influence for you, your children, and those you encounter. Random and intentional acts of kindness are golden nuggets, as there is no better way to quickly raise your vibration.

This positive energy is what gives you momentum to create the future you want with your children. The ability to have control of your thoughts helps declutter your mind, opening space to receive inspiration and ideas. Listen to your intuition—to what your body is telling you. Continue to make subtle shifts in your daily lifestyle with conscious intentions, acts of kindness, and positive thoughts, and eliminate gossip and talking behind people's backs, negative thoughts, and exaggeration. Focused and continued personal development will always keep you moving in fast forward. As you become open to receiving the little messages from the universe (that you already have inside you), you will see people and experiences in your path guiding and moving you closer to the future you visualized.

Happy Place

Everyone needs a happy place! The beauty of its creation is that you can tap into it anytime, no matter where you are, because this place is in your imagination. A bonus is that as you grow and expand, so can your happy place. Think of it this way—it is like watching a movie on the screen of your mind. And you are the creator, director, and producer. Personally, I have several of them! This strategic visualization tool can be used when you start to feel anxious, nervous, fearful, doubtful, or frustrated. This is a practice in awareness by "catching" these feelings as soon as possible.

For many people, negative feelings are their baseline. They get consumed and entangled by negative feelings, which ultimately leads to poor decisions.

This recycling of unwanted thoughts, spiraling, and even making stuff up that has not even happened yet is not a good place to be. Remember: your mind is powerful. How you choose to use that power is up to you. The more negative energy you feed it, the more it festers and escalates. When you stay in this state, you have successfully blocked your energy flow, leaving you feeling stuck and making it almost impossible to reflect on the situation and move forward. The opposite holds true as well. The more positive, yummy stuff you feed your mind, the more you exude optimism, clarity, and grace. Everyone around you sees it and feels it. That's why it is crucial that when it feels like you're spiraling out of control like a tornado, you simply visit your happy place.

Going to your happy place is a habit, and like all habits, it needs to be developed. Trust that you will feel better when you go there. It's just like going to the gym—getting there is the hard part, but once you do get there, you're good. Your happy place is a form of release, building mental strength and helping you to feel better. You are working your mental muscle! Know that just like muscle memory, cells have memories of your past, and it takes work to shift the old energy and release your conditioned beliefs to manage your emotions.

Take your time and enjoy the creation! Trust in the process. This one tool may take days to complete, but it is worth it. The mind and body now have a blueprint for a most rejuvenating mindset. As with implementing any new habit, repetition and consistency are the cornerstones. Be patient—you are taking care of something incredible—your mind.

Once you master this tool, recognize that you are modeling your power to choose your thoughts for your family. Your children hear your words, see your actions, and learn your behaviors. They follow your lead. You are clearing the path for them, and when the time is right, you can lead your children to create their own happy place. Invite others with empowering language to create the belief that they are the creators, directors, and producers of their own lives.

You are always free to better manage your emotions with visualization by:

- Applying your happy place tool to "catch" unwanted feelings.
- Pausing with intention to transition to your happy place, managing unwanted emotions before they escalate.
- Having gratitude for pulling yourself out of an unwanted space, taking back your power from your mind.
- Mindfully going inside to manage your feelings and actions.
- Avoiding outside "solutions" like food, alcohol, slamming doors, or yelling.

Forward Vision

You learned that you have control over your thoughts and that mental strength can only be achieved through practice. Forward vision thinkers strive to move on to create their best lives. Creative energy thinking and spiritual practices help you slow down and accomplish what is important to you. Forward vision thinkers also do not use their past or current circumstances to hold them back.

If we want to be free, we must stop locking ourselves into the prison of our pasts. Every moment can be an open door to new adventures, but only you can decide to walk through for yourself. Worry less about the unexpected. Yes, get up, get grateful, and get in sync with who you want to be. You can't go back and change the past, so start where you are and change the future instead.

Every day brings choices to envision your future. It all begins with awareness of how you want to feel in this moment. Ask yourself, *do I want...*

- Stress or Peace?
- Annoyance or Calmness?
- Negativity or Positivity?
- Frustration or Satisfaction?

- Hate or Love?
- Heartlessness or Compassion?
- Anger or Happiness?
- Fear or Faith?
- Despair or Hope?
- Worry or Harmony?
- Sadness or Joy?

Each is your choice to make when visualizing your future.

Vision Board

Vision boards are great tools for forward thinkers. They capture your visualizations in very real ways, enabling you to physically see where you want to go in the future.

Why create a vision board? Some reasons include:

- You are ready to make a shift to reinvent, declare, and claim the life path your heart truly desires.
- You want to ignite that spark of internal motivation, allowing inspiration to take action.
- You are ready for self-discovery, awareness, and consciousness to reconnect with yourself.
- You expect to rise and thrive, exploring your potential and finding purpose.

Create your vision board with a mindset for inspiration and exploration. When deciding which items to post on your vision board, make sure:

- It brings a huge smile to your face.
- It makes you feel empowered and motivated.
- It makes you feel excited and scared at the same time—this is when you know you have a great goal!

- You know you do not have to have it all figured out to move forward.
- You stand in front of your vision board at least twice per day. Personally, I brush my teeth while standing in front of my vision board every morning and before bed. I have an electric toothbrush and it goes for two minutes. Look at it. Read the words and phrases. Let your mind expand on the pictures.
- Expect your dreams and goals to form. Picture yourself already living your dream and attaining your goal(s).
- Be bold. Hang your vision board in a place for others to see. This will invite conversation and empower others to create their own vision boards. Share your excitement.
- Each time you engage with your vision board, you are giving energy to your dreams and goals, allowing more feelings and emotions to emerge, and gaining momentum for you to take action.

I Ask My True Self

- *Where is my happy place?*
- *What brings a smile to my face?*
- *What makes me feel free inside?*
- *What do I want to achieve, be, do, or have in my life?*
- *What pictures will I look for?*
- *What date will my vision board be completed?*
- *How can I involve my child in the process?*
- *How can I encourage my child to create their own vision board with my help?*

Aligning Thoughts with Actions

Set a future-thinking goal. If you don't know how, ask yourself:

- What does my heart desire?

- What puts a smile on my face?
- What makes me feel good?
- What makes me happy?
- What makes me wake up eager to start my day?

Visualize meeting this goal. Visualize it with as much detail as if you were watching it play out as a movie on a big screen. You don't have to know how you're going to get there. In fact, we rarely do. But that's not our job. Ask yourself, *how does this "movie" make me feel?* The next steps include:

- Setting a due date. Write it on your calendar. A goal without a due date is simply a dream.
- Sharing it with others. The more you talk about your goals and dreams, the more energy you give them.
- Remembering your worth. Know you are worthy of the good you desire.
- Staying committed and being consistent. Commitment and consistency are key to this practice.

Try some of these random acts of kindness to kick up your future-thinking vibe! If you do any of these random acts of kindness, you will feel good for being kind and the receiver will be happy and may be more apt to do the same for someone else. Can you see the ripple effect?

- When leaving a breakfast place, say "Enjoy your breakfast" in passing as someone else is entering.
- Whenever you buy a book, buy two or three and then give the extras away.
- Call or text someone today and tell them how awesome they are.
- Check in with someone you know who is struggling.
- Send someone a card in the mail listing all the great things you love about them.

- Pay for the coffee order of the person in line behind you.
- When a server goes the extra mile in their service, or if you can see they are having a difficult day (they are new on the job or covering extra tables), take notice and show kindness—leave a larger tip or write something nice on the receipt.
- Volunteer to be involved in a community fundraiser or charity.
- Give a compliment to a family member and take it deeper by saying why.
- Try doing something nice for someone who annoys you.
- When you're at the gym and someone runs in late to class, help them set up.

Improve the energy in your home to help support your child, so that they feel safe. Let's focus on the child's bedroom space:

1. Make the child's bedroom as comfortable as possible.
2. Create a space in which the child feels safe.
3. Avoid any anger or raising your voice or showing any signs of negative energies while in your child's bedroom.
4. Avoid using the bedroom as some kind of punishment tool, as this does not create a sense of safety.
5. Declutter as much of the space as possible. Too much clutter feels chaotic, and this energy could be reflected in the child's behavior.
6. When in the child's bedroom, be as calm as possible, with a positive energy, speaking softly and slowly.
7. Before bed, turn off and unplug all electrical devices in the room and anything else which may be emitting EMFs (electric and magnetic fields). Or place devices in flight mode.
8. Try to keep as much air flowing through the room as possible. Open windows when you can and when it is safe to do so, to help remove any negative energy that may be trapped within the room.

9. To help raise the energy, try using pure essential oils in a diffuser. (This is assuming there are no allergies. Follow safety guidelines, and check with your physician before using any new substance. Some essential oils may not be recommended for small children under a certain age.)
10. Avoid using artificial air fresheners or fragrances of any kind, as this can create the opposite of the desired effect.

Tips for envisioning your happy place:

1. Ask yourself these questions:
   a. Where are you?
   b. Are you outside?
   c. What are you wearing?
   d. What do you see next to you?
   e. What do you see in the distance?
   f. Is it windy?
   g. Are there clouds?
   h. Flowers? A rainbow? Mountains?
   i. Is it raining?
   j. What are you doing?
   k. Are you laughing, singing, dancing, running?
   l. Are there any pets, food, or beverages involved?
   m. Who is with you?
   n. Are you touching anything?
   o. Do you smell anything? Flowers? Fresh cut grass? Popcorn or other foods?
   p. How does it make you feel?
   q. How can you make this place more special and fun?
2. Include as many of the five senses as you can in the description of your happy place. What words come to mind when you go to this happy

place? Create this space with as much description and feeling as possible. You should feel free and feel that the image in your mind of what you desire is real. Then you will be instantly transported to a better place of calmness and joy. Do a body scan in your happy place. Are your shoulders relaxed? Is your jaw relaxed? How about your belly?

3. Use colored markers or colored paper. Write your name or the words "My Happy Place" at the top. Maybe use card stock paper and put it in a protective sheet cover, frame it, or write it in your journal. Look at it every night before going to sleep and every morning when you wake up. The more you visualize your happy place, the more it becomes imprinted on the screen of your mind. You are building new brain cells for your happy place. It will become automatic as this new, positive habit is established. Give yourself permission to change it when you see fit, inviting more ways to think deeper in more details and with more action.
4. Next, record yourself reading the description of your happy place. Listening to the recording in your own voice establishes a connection, developing trust with your own voice and words.
5. Be creative. Look for opportunities to share your happy place with your child, family, and friends, as this is how your place will magnify, allowing even more energy and inspiration. You are the movie star of this unique safe space you can visit for peace of mind whenever life gets wild and crazy. Remember, it organically keeps expanding and changing as your interests change.
6. See yourself in that place. See yourself smiling, happy, relaxed, comfortable, safe, and doing something you enjoy.

Reflections of Visualization . . .

The future belongs to those who believe in the beauty of their dreams.

~ Eleanor Roosevelt

Reflections of Visualization . . .

Creative Visualization is a spiritual exercise using your thoughts and imagination to change your life in a positive way.

~ Meryl Hershey Beck

Chapter 6

The Art of Communication

It's Not Just the Words We Say

Positive Affirmation

Today I will communicate positively and listen with my heart.

Sharing in the Extraordinary Journey

~ Patrice Headd, M.Ed., Special Education, Preschool Teacher

One sweet little boy who struggles with anxiety came to school one day and shared with me he was very scared about going to kindergarten registration. We talked about how ready he was and how much fun it would be in his new school. The day after the kindergarten registration, he told me it was hard, but he remembered to use his power words, "I can do hard things." As he shared his experience, his eyes lit up. I could see the pride he was feeling with this major accomplishment and the emotional strength he himself had been able to build with positive affirmations. This five-year-old taught me a lesson that day. Simple routines that we can easily incorporate into our daily life can make an enormous difference in our mindset, behavior, and results! I will be forever grateful for this sweet little boy with his giant heart.

~ Heidi Rome, Mom and Bestselling Author of *You Just Have to Love Me: Drawing Strength from the Unseen*

One of the pitfalls of this journey is that we buy into the tragedy narrative around autism and believe that it is our role as a "good mother" to "fix" our "broken" child. We go to great lengths and great expense to explore "healing" alternatives and interventions in our desperate attempt to make our child be (or at least look) "normal" for others. At the heart of our extreme actions is the fear that we are letting our child down and we are bad mothers if we don't make this autism thing stop ruining his life. The problem here is that we can be so consumed with the idea of changing our child that we forget to accept and love them unconditionally for who they are. Driven by fear, we make decisions about our child that are based on whether it fulfills our limitless need to be a "good mother" and not on whether it is what our child himself needs and wants here and now. We make it about us, not about them.

I'll give you an example. I had gone into my autistic son's school to work on his communication skills with him. To keep the practice conversation interesting and relevant to Ethan, the teacher asked what we did everyday outside of school. The truth was that every waking moment before and after school and on weekends was spent on a therapy or an activity related to addressing the symptoms or deficits associated with autism. I launched into a litany of the current interventions we were doing—physical therapy, occupational therapy, speech therapy, yoga for special children, Chinese medicine, supplements, acupressure, Tomatis listening therapy, Brain Gym, homeopathy, methyl B12 injections. I also proudly rattled off the ones we were considering (hyperbaric pressure chamber therapy, micromovement therapy in San Francisco, stem cell transplantation in Panama, swimming with dolphins in Belarus). The list was endless, and I was aware of a self-soothing, but frantic voice in my head as I was speaking to the stunned teacher. *You're a good mother. You're a good mother. Keep doing all this and it'll be OK.*

In the middle of my frantic soliloquy, Ethan reached toward the letterboard, his pointer finger outstretched. To my shock and horror, he spelled out his response to my words: "I am tired." I will admit to you that I resisted at first. "Ethan, buddy, you need all this. It's to help you." Yet, I could not unsee what he had urgently communicated to me. I remembered suddenly what I had dismissed—his physical therapist telling me that Ethan would sometimes lie down and close his eyes in the middle of a game or obstacle course. I felt faint as I realized how exhausted he must be . . . and had no other way to tell me besides behavior I had refused to understand and listen to. Within a week, I began to cut back on some of Ethan's activities and handpicked which ones to keep. His overall behavior did improve, and he calmed down a bit as he rested more. Most of all, though, I realized I had time to just enjoy being with my son. I took back my role as his loving mom and took away his burdensome status as my project.

Think about it. If your child is overbooked with therapy after therapy, the message he is likely receiving is, *I am broken. Mommy is very unhappy that I am broken, and I need to go to all these different experts to fix me. I am not okay as I am.*

I chose to focus on my child's wonderful qualities, including his differences, and celebrate the pleasure he brings me. This is powerful therapy, for him and for me. Unconditional love and acceptance have the most healing impact of anything else I've ever tried. That's saying a lot!

I Grow My Wisdom

The ability to communicate effectively is one of life's most valuable skills. It is the way in which we connect with others and build relationships. How we communicate is a part of who we are at our core. The words you consciously choose can be incredibly powerful, either in a positive way or in a negative one. But the more positive, loving, and empowering words you speak daily, the more you and others around you will feel those emotions.

When we talk about communication, many automatically think about the words they speak. However, that's only half of it. The other half of communication is how we listen. But many also mistakenly believe that listening means hearing. The difference? We hear with our ears, and we listen with our hearts. Listening is a skill that allows deeper connections between you and the person with whom you're in a conversation.

Someone can be speaking right in front of us, and often, our thoughts are running wild with "mind chatter." We hear their words, but with our minds preoccupied, we do not have the ability to correlate those words with their proper meaning. Most of the time, we don't even realize we are hearing, but not listening. How often are we doing this with our children?

Our children observe what we're doing. And they hear us, even when we don't think they do. Release your expectations and be open to the unexpected. Know with confidence that your actions are being observed and your words are being heard, so choose them wisely.

My suggestion is to make communication with your child fun in as many ways as possible. Practice with them and with the rest of your family, or even at work and the store—there are opportunities everywhere to sharpen communication skills. Try the "Call Out" game. Have everyone in the house call you out when you use a negative word, and then use another word to make it positive. I promise you, this will change the dynamic of how your family speaks with each other.

For example, if you say, "I am so frustrated with the computer; I never can do this right," your child picks up on the words, body language, and tone, and no doubt feels your negative energy. When this happens, use it as a teaching moment. When your child calls you out, say thank you for pointing it out and work together to figure out alternative words that could be more positive. If your child does not pick up on it, bring it to their attention and ask them for help in choosing better words. You are also recognizing their value and contribution, which builds your child's self-esteem.

To expand on the example above, say, "I am really thankful I have a computer; not everyone has one." Then say something positive like, "Every day I am getting better and better at using the computer. I am reading the prompts better and will Google how to do this next time."

Every word we speak holds light and energy, and that energy ripples to everyone we encounter—our children, our spouses, our co-workers. Children with autism are tuned into the energy of others, as they rely on their senses to communicate and understand much more than we do. When one's energy does not equate to one's words, they feel it instantaneously and know it is not authentic.

This role modeling with your words, always looking for the good in any situation and appreciating what you have, creates a more positive experience for your children. It also demonstrates what you can do next time ("I am reading the prompts better and will Google how to do this") to keep yourself from escalating into deeper frustration. This is the power of communication.

Feel the richness of this communication habit today. Apply this example to any situation to keep your energy grounded. Yes, energy shifts with negative words, just like it does with a negative attitude. Look at it this way—we are either thinking low thoughts or we are thinking high thoughts. And your words directly impact your energy. Clear intentions with elevated emotions give energy to either your wanted or unwanted words, so choose consciously and wisely, giving the right energy to your desired outcome.

In another example, instead of saying, "It makes me so mad when you leave dirty dishes in the sink," try saying, "It makes me so happy when you rinse and put your dishes in the dishwasher." They both are making the same point. Try it. Say one and see how it makes you feel. Say the other and see how it makes you feel. The first phrase puts the child on the defensive; they feel they are disappointing you or didn't do it right or that their effort was not good enough. The other makes them feel worthy, good, helpful, and appreciated.

Liberation happens when you realize that you are complaining, criticizing, commiserating, or exaggerating, and you catch yourself and stop. Remember—progress over perfection. Learn to pause and think before you speak. Ask yourself, "Does this help me get to my goal?" Place reminders around the house. Maybe paint on various rocks the words *pause*, *kindness*, *create*, or *love*, and keep them in common areas. Visualizations around our home help those thoughts penetrate deeper into our subconscious, helping us retrain our minds and, by extension, our communication skills.

The Power of Autosuggestion

Autosuggestion is a tool for reprogramming your subconscious mind. It is a method of planting your precise desires inside your subconscious—a deliberate intention to make a change. It is a practice with the mindset of believing that you have already succeeded, and it is a form of communication. Autosuggestion is practiced in the present tense. You have the trust and the faith that you will become this change. You are learning to foster a belief with focused energy, creating change, allowing inspiration and action, and achieving more of what you desire. What do we all want? Peace, happiness, balance, and joy for ourselves and for all.

As you continue to master this technique, you are role modeling and sharing these tools with your children and those around you, showing them how to build an epic mindset! When the time is right, you can encourage your children to think about a goal or a habit they want to improve and come up with a list of autosuggestions together.

One way to make autosuggestion fun with your child is to pour a thin layer of sugar on a baking sheet. Your child writes a positive a word or phrase about themselves, like "I am strong" in the sugar and says it out loud. Then, shake the baking sheet and write the next one. This will add a texture component to increase reprogramming of the thoughts in your child's mind about himself or herself. You can also take wax paper and dump some chocolate pudding onto it and write the affirmation in the pudding with a finger, and then wipe it off and write the next one. This will make the activity more interactive, fun, and yummy!

Listen with Your Heart

Truly listening with our hearts is a life skill that allows for deeper connections. Yet, mind chatter often prevents us from doing so. But to communicate effectively, we must listen. Start by becoming more aware of the issue. Pay attention to see how often you are fully present when communicating with your children or anyone, for that matter. And how often you're not. When we are thinking about a million other things, we cannot be present for the person right in front of us. We cannot concentrate and focus while distracted by never-ending racing thoughts.

Now, that is not to say that you should be interrupted at any time the other person (including your child) deems acceptable. If you are in the middle of something and someone starts talking, try saying, "Please give me a minute to wrap this up. You deserve my undivided attention. I want to hear all about what you want to tell me!"

I have learned that our children are our greatest teachers when we truly listen to what they have to say. Make the conscious decision to listen with your heart. Recognize that people want to be heard and commit to being present with the person with whom you are communicating. Try listening to understand and not listening to reply. This is very different. One of the best things we can understand is that people just want to know that they are valued. They want to hear the words, "I hear you."

Try it! The results will be all you need to make a change!

I Ask My True Self

- *Did I say something to someone that was not nice?*
- *How could I have worded it differently?*
- *What change do I want to make today?*

- *What do I want more of in my life?*
- *What are twenty positive affirmations or autosuggestion phrases for something I want to change?*
- *Whom do I connect with and why?*
- *Whom do I disconnect with and why?*

Aligning Thoughts with Actions

Lisa Drennan (MERGE Diverse Abilities Inclusion Consulting; Let's Get to Success Approach, Exclusion to Inclusion) gives the following valuable advice when it comes to communication:

> When giving a direction, instruction, or request, be mindful to phrase it in the "positive." In other words, frame your statement to focus on what you'd like to occur rather than pointing out that something is being done wrong or that your child is acting badly. For example, if you are visiting your local pool and your child enthusiastically starts to run on the pool deck, excited to get to the stairs and get in, instead of saying "no running," you would simply say "walk please."

Other examples include:

Instead of this . . .	**Say this . . .**
You're not listening! I said don't leave your LEGOs scattered on the floor.	Please look around and pick up any LEGOs from the floor and put them in the container.
Stop interrupting me, or you are not going to have computer time.	If you wait until I'm off the phone to talk to me, you will be able to have computer time tonight.
Don't talk so loudly, or we are going to have to leave the library.	When we are in the library, we use our inside voices.

Forming your statements in the positive provides an opportunity to teach and reinforce appropriate or expected interactions. You are also role modeling for them positive problem-solving techniques by using this more positive way of interacting with them.

Tips for using autosuggestion with the strategic step-by-step creative energy thinking process:

1. Clearly decide what you want. What does your heart desire? It can be a habit you want to change or a desire for a better self-image, self-confidence, or self-esteem. It can be optimal health, healing, forgiveness, or a better career, home, or vacation. It can be anything you want to be, do, or have!
2. Declare a conscious intention of the desired change and write it down.
3. Write a list of twenty autosuggestions in the present tense, as if you have already succeeded in your desire, even if you don't believe it right now. Embrace and reinforce positive words. For example, *I am experiencing optimal health with joy and ease. I celebrate my strong immune system. I never get sick. I am having fun while exercising my body. I am strong, fit, and attractive.*
4. Visualize each autosuggestion. Imagine a picture in each autosuggestion, depicting you already achieving your goal and what that looks like.
5. Make a commitment to write each morning and evening for thirty to sixty days, reading and visualizing your autosuggestion list. Always keep a journal nearby during this practice, as it allows you to write any thoughts or ideas that come to mind or actions to take. They will come!
6. Practice reading your list with intention. Each day, allow more feeling and expansion of your thoughts and visualizations of each autosuggestion. You create that image and into the subconscious mind it goes. We are putting it there deliberately.
7. Record it on your phone through the video option. Try putting your hand on your heart while saying your autosuggestions, making a deeper connection. I listen to my autosuggestions in the car on Bluetooth.

8. Know with certainty that you have attained it. Have faith. You are not doing this alone. It is already done. When you believe in this way, it is much easier to let go of resistance and the change naturally occurs. Trust. Believe you are the desired change already. We become what we think.

Tips for listening with your heart:

- Take a breath, intentionally clear your mind of chatter, judgment, and resistance, and be present.
- Embrace the attitude that you recognize this person is worthy of your undivided attention.
- Desire to listen to everything they want to share with you.
- Focus on the person right in front of you; put your cell phone aside and make eye contact.
- Feel their words.
- Notice the other person's body language.
- Rest your hand on your heart space to deepen the connection.
- Add a light touch from your hand to theirs, or a touch to the shoulder if it feels right.
- Offer inspiration and support.
- Cherish this moment, as you will never be in this moment ever again. Be grateful. So many people regret not truly listening or hearing the person right in front of them. You can never get the moment back. Don't miss the opportunity to listen with your heart.
- Be authentic. You will never win in life by trying to be someone you are not.
- Allow the other person to speak their thought(s). Avoid interrupting.
- If you find yourself in judgment, STOP. They do feel your energy.
- Observation is power. Judgment is weakness.

Reflections of Communication . . .

Listen with the intent to understand, not the intent to reply.

~ Stephen Covey

Reflections of Communication . . .

You have to learn to say no without feeling guilty. Setting boundaries is healthy. You need to learn to respect and take care of yourself.

~ Unknown

Chapter 7

Body Scan

Activate Your Blueprint to Rejuvenation

Positive Affirmation

Today I will honor my body and what it is trying to tell me.

Sharing in the Extraordinary Journey

~ Colleen Duggan-Cuomo, the Yogi

First, I pay attention to their breath—focus on the exhale, as this is when relaxation begins. I'll say softly, "Now with every exhale, think of melting, relaxing, and letting go." I cue this on the exhale because of the physiological effects (as well as how our respiratory system works). When we exhale, our nervous system is allowed to relax. I guide them to become aware of just that one feeling. I ask them to feel the difference, feel the quality of the inhale versus the quality of the exhale.

Once they are feeling their breath settle in, I can see their bodies begin to relax physically—from how they sit, to where their shoulders are, to their facial expressions. Next, I invite them to start feeling a heaviness in their body, so the relaxation deepens. I guide them to notice where they feel heaviness, twitches, aches, and restlessness, and tell them to give themselves permission to let it all go.

As I see they are ready, I visually have them move through their body relaxing, specifically the jaw, eyes, across the forehead, teeth, lips, face, cheeks, and nose. Now, it's time to invite in the awareness that since they have relaxed their bodies, they can now relax their minds. I invite them to continue to use their breath to guide themselves deeper into relaxation.

Sometimes, my students become distracted at the end of class. My suggestion is to listen to the sound of their breath (breathing loud in and out with audible exhales)—a great way to get back to relaxation for those who are soothed by sound. Relaxing the body and the mind is potent and powerful for the nervous system. I see the results and benefits from body scans every time we do these in class. This is magic for these children!

~ Nicole Dauz, Mom and Founder of SelfCare4Caregivers

Conscious breathing is one of my top three self-care tips that I share with caregivers. It's something that we can do at any moment, and we can control the length of time that we need to do it in order to calm us down or reset the moment.

It's one of the activities that Summer and I do together to reset and move from a place of frustration to peace. I have her sit on my lap, wrap her legs around my waist and her arms around my neck and we do deep breaths together, as I count out loud. Even though she resists at first, usually after 30 seconds, I can feel her body relax and she starts to breathe with me.

After we're done, we always touch noses (our special connection thing), and we walk away calm, peaceful, and ready for the next activity. Never underestimate the power of taking five minutes to take deep breaths and show your body that it's safe.

~ Dr. Elizabeth Joy Shaffer, Mom and Therapist

Plowing through fear for us parents raising children with autism can be challenging. We are constantly feeling pulled to drop everything and tend to our child's needs instantly. We worry and doubt ourselves about whether we are doing enough, thinking we should be doing more, which leaves us feeling exhausted, depleted, and stressed. Our mind is conditioned that everyone's time comes first with a fear of not being a good mother if we take time for ourselves. Setting boundaries for yourself (time for yourself) to rest and reset takes a mindset modification. Our mindset controls our actions .

If we believe that when we are taking this time for ourselves, it is helping our children and us, we are much more likely to follow through. Implementing a new self-care habit is an act of self-love, and it is needed to show up as the best version of ourselves. This means taking a break to go to our happy place, meditate, read, listen to music, walk in the park, or just sit each day for at least ten minutes. But as you may have experienced before, when we step away for a moment, something can happen that confirms to our subconscious that we must always be there, and we are the only ones who can handle our children's needs. Here is where mindset comes in. Having faith and trust that others can help and be there for our kids as they need them to be while we are not there is such a great gift to you and your child. And teaching your child to have patience and the need for quiet time is a wonderful lesson. When you start to take this time, you may find your children trying to steal back this time from you. If you are in your room resting or meditating and your child comes in the room, say in a low, calm voice, "This quiet time makes me feel good, so I need to take these ten minutes, and when I do, I will have so much energy to come and play with you!"

I Grow My Wisdom

What Is a Body Scan?

A body scan is a tool used to notice the different sensations in the body, without any judgment or labeling, guiding both your body and mind into a state of rejuvenation simply and effectively. It is an invitation to experience each body part. Often, people are unaware that their muscles are in a state of contraction or restriction, and for some, this becomes their baseline, which sets the stage for a closed, cramped, congested, crowded space in the physical body as well as the mind.

Daily body scans help you feel grounded, relaxed, present, and connected to your body by allowing creative energy to flow more easily. With a body scan, you can detect blockages and work to dissolve them. It generates a keener awareness of your body in the moment. It also helps to reduce anxiety, improve sleep, and manage pain by tapping into the body for a better connection. Simply, body scans bring loving kindness and appreciation to the body. We demand so much from our bodies and can be so judgmental, neglectful, and disconnected. We deserve a break.

The objective of a body scan is to bring awareness to your body and consciously release any physical restrictions. Yes, that word again! *Awareness!* Awareness is the cornerstone of all that we do. Awareness is being free to be you. Make a daily habit during a certain time of day to release tension before it escalates physically or mentally into uneasiness, anxiety, or physical pain in the form of a stomachache, headache, restlessness, loss of appetite, exhaustion, or moodiness.

This tool can be practiced anytime, anywhere, at work or before sleep. Body scans can last a few minutes or for as long as you desire. There are both long and short variations, so that you can navigate your entire body or select only certain body parts. You can use a meditation app to find guided body scans, or you can bring yourself through a body scan yourself, as needed.

Breathing

Breathing more deeply energizes your body and mood, almost like magic. Deep breaths immediately fill you with calmness, while detoxing your body. Most of our breathing is regulated automatically, while conscious breathing allows you to discover new ways of shifting your energy and perception.

Conscious breathing can and should be done anytime and anywhere. Do it often! Practice until it becomes a habit—the more you get connected with your breath, the more your body and mind will thank you for these treats of replenishing fresh air. You can change your energy instantly by taking deep breaths, which bring more tranquility and a lightness of being.

Whether you are put on the spot, unexpectedly running late to an appointment, or feeling stressed, simply use the wonders of your breath. Take a long deep breath, then call and let the person know your status. No long story, no big explanation. Be appreciative of their understanding. Do not assume what the person is thinking—that only wastes valuable energy. Choose to listen to some soothing music, your positive autosuggestions, or go to your happy place, where you can reset your mindset. The traffic you are in is out of your control. But the way you react to the traffic *is* in your control.

Trust in the process of expansion of the breath and how it affects your body and mind. When you have time, incorporate conscious breathing as an activity by gently closing your eyes and simply witnessing your breath as it flows in and out. Inhale through the nose and exhale through the mouth. Invite the other senses into this moment. Gently place your hand on the belly or chest and observe it rise and fall.

Now, allow yourself to be totally in sync with life. Be present. If you are outside, take a moment and really look around, see the beauty, soak up all that life has to offer, raising your eyes and heart to the sky. Then, close your eyes and just listen with your open heart as the sounds of life sing their song to you. Maybe place a hand over your heart to deepen the connection. What sounds are you hearing? Birds, wind, squirrels in the trees, chipmunks racing around, raindrops hitting leaves on the ground, cars, voices, leaves rustling, wind chimes, a woodpecker? If you venture indoors, then listen to and hear your breath, and maybe play some recorded nature sounds or soft relaxing music.

In this way, you are increasing your consciousness. Invite a long, deep breath, and maybe try holding it for three to five seconds. In this moment, while holding your breath, allow your body complete stillness. Nothing is moving except the beating of your heart. Then, with awareness, release what doesn't serve your body. It may be aches, pains, sadness, or worry.

As you breathe in through the nose, notice if the air feels cool or warm. Maybe try blocking one nostril and see what you notice. This is a simple yet energy-changing game you can play with your child that will reinforce a conscious breathing habit. Their eyes can be opened or closed. Their bodies and minds will love the increased flow of oxygen and blood flow bathing each and every cell in love, leaving you refreshed and with the knowledge that everything will be okay.

Our actions are a model for our kids on how to perform. Showing them that you are taking these moments, a block of time for yourself to have more energy and a clear mind to be with them, shows them how to listen to, and stand up for, what their body and mind needs in order to be healthy. So, permit yourself to release your fears and resistance to taking time for yourself. Also, when taking these moments, make sure not to carry thoughts of worry, doubt, anxiety, and uncertainty, so both your body and mind can have the peaceful break they deserve.

Breaking through Fear

Once you understand the idea that your fears and doubts are based on recycled past experiences and beliefs of others that have been impressed upon your mind (maybe since you were a child), you will have the ability to plow through your fear and doubt on demand. Understand that nothing will change until you change your paradigm. We believe these things, even though they may not be true at all. We have been conditioned to think that we can't do something, or that we are not good enough or smart enough. Many of us go through life accepting what others put into our minds. We literally believe it and let these early criticisms hold us back. If you accept the idea that you are fearful and have self-doubt in certain things, you will continue that path of believing it. The longer you believe an idea, the more it reinforces those images in your mind.

There are three basic types of fear: Phobias, "what ifs," and the immediate "fight-or-flight" response. The most destructive fear is the "what ifs" because it is based on speculation. The mind is paralyzed by continually analyzing scenarios of what may or may not happen, and there are infinite possibilities. Fear is debilitating. It distorts perception and blocks rational thoughts and higher reasoning.

Once you recognize that your fear-based limiting thoughts are only in your mind, then you can stop fearful limiting thoughts with conscious awareness and reprogramming. Inviting thoughts of "I can" and "Why not me?" and "I can do anything I set my mind to" give you the new mindset of success, limitlessness, and desire! This is where the tool of autosuggestion is a game changer. As you know, the subconscious mind accepts anything you put into it. Mastery of your thoughts is what you are allowing to enter your mind.

Think of a tall, clear container filled with water with sand stuck at the bottom. Visualize the container as your mind or body. Imagine pouring more clean water into the container, which represents filling yourself with a positive mindset. As you fill your container daily with positive intentions, your happy place, autosuggestions, gratitude, meditation, and acts of kindness, along with eating healthier and increasing your movement, the sand begins to lift and swirl around, and it probably gets a little muddy for a while. After a couple of months of pouring goodness into the container daily, the muddy sand rises higher toward the top, and eventually, the muddy sand spills out of the container and your mind and body are left with all the clean, revitalizing, refreshing water! You are consciously transforming your container by filling it up with all the good, yummy stuff. You are now enjoying the benefits of a lighter, cleaner, refreshed container that has been replenished and reclaimed!

I Ask My True Self

- *How do I want to show up for myself and others?*
- *What do I want to radiate out into the world?*
- *How can I benefit from the wonders of the breath tool?*
- *How is my body physically feeling in this moment?*
- *How could daily body scans benefit me?*
- *What if I applied this tool proactively, knowing of a situation that may cause my body to shut down, tighten, and react rather than respond?*
- *When would I use this tool?*

Aligning Thoughts with Actions

Try the Energy Changer Game

- Set a timer for one minute.
- For that one minute, follow this breathing technique:
  - As you breathe in, hold your breath for three to five seconds and then exhale.
  - Think about or recite positive words that resonate with you (I breathe in trust and exhale fear; I breathe in love and abundance and exhale anger and lack; I breathe in confidence and certainty and exhale resistance and doubt).
  - With each breath feel all aspects of your being—mind, body, and spirit— become open, spacious, and free.
  - Know with certainty you are rejuvenating every part of your body.
- REPEAT for one minute or longer as desired.

Try one of these Body Scans and explore the rejuvenation:

- Bring your attention to each body part. Notice how it feels; then consciously breathe into that body part, breathing in joy and hope. Exhale and release any doubt and fear until your body softens and feels better. Let your breath untie the knots in your body and mind.
- Bring your attention to your eyes, ears, and mouth. Rest your hands on your eyes, recognizing the good that you see. Then bring your hands to rest on your ears with awareness of everything you hear, and listen with your heart. Finally, bring your hands to your lips as a reminder to speak kind words today.
- Bring your attention to each body part and squeeze, clench, tighten up that part as much as you can, and hold the squeeze for five seconds; then release the muscle completely. As you travel to each body part, visualize as you inhale a deep, long breath that you are filling up a red balloon, and as you exhale, watch the balloon float away, taking away what doesn't serve your body. Begin with the forehead and travel down to the eyes, cheeks, jaw, neck, arms, hands, chest, belly, buttocks, thighs, calves, feet, and toes. Customize as desired to make this practice shorter or longer.
- Bring your attention to the top of your head. Visualize any clutter and negative thoughts leaping out of your mind into a river, floating down and over a waterfall and just disappearing.
- Bring your attention to your forehead. Feel your wrinkles gently smooth out any worries, allowing for softness.
- Bring your attention to your eyes. Visualize the muscles behind your eyes melting like ice cubes in warm water.
- Bring your attention to your jaw. Let it rest. (There is a lot of physical activity with the jaw from chewing to saying things you regret or holding in words.) Bring your tongue to the roof of your mouth. This action is known to be a natural tranquilizer for the nervous system and reduces tension.

- Bring your attention to your shoulders. Lift your shoulders up and back letting your shoulder blades slide down. Visualize lifting heavy loads of frustration, junk from the past, and stressors in the moment and gently throwing them into a fire and watching them burn and disintegrate. Feel the shoulders lighten and move more freely.
- Bring attention to your arms. Allow them to float by your side, maybe with your palms face up ready to receive goodness, peace, and joy, or palms facing down if you're searching for connectivity, balance, or to become more grounded.
- Bring your attention to your belly. Feel the belly rise and fall with each breath. Visualize standing on the beach and the sun beaming down, bathing you in warmth, and notice how the light reflects off the ocean saltwater, putting a smile on your face. Allow your belly to rise and fall with the ebb and flow of the ocean waves drifting in and out. Feel a warm wave of relaxation and comfort wash over your body.
- Bring your attention to your hips. Feel them open and release any negative emotions that are stuck. Visualize black clouds of rooted emotions flowing out of your hips into thin air, leaving you with massive amounts of space and extra flexibility in your gait.
- Bring your attention to your back. Visualize a ball of light heating up, centered on your lower back, loosening your muscles and nerves, sending messages of healing light up your spinal column, feeling at ease with flexibility and comfort.
- Bring your attention to your legs. Visualize yourself immersed in an outdoor pool, as your body is gently bobbing in cleansing, refreshing water in a dreamy state, and your legs feel light, rejuvenated, and playful.
- Bring your attention to your feet. Visualize strong roots from the soles of your feet, feeling grounded and supported, traveling deep into the earth and attaching firmly. Visualize Mother Earth's nutrients, light, and warmth from the sun, moon, stars, and other galaxies streaming through the soles of your feet, bringing bright, healing light to every cell, fiber, and nerve, bathing your body in love.

You now hold the power to customize a body scan of your own! This practice can also be extremely useful for parenting your children. Use it before (and, as needed, during) transitions and events that have the potential to cause them anxiety. Use it to calm their fear-based beliefs. It is also a powerful and engaging tool for teachers to implement in the classroom.

Reflections of the Body . . .

Master your breath, let the self be in bliss, contemplate on the sublime within you.

~ Tirumalai Krishnamacharya

Reflections of the Body . . .

Yoga is the perfect opportunity to be curious about who you are.

~ Jason Crandell

Chapter 8

Connecting Your Body & Soul

The Power of Meditation & Yoga

Positive Affirmation

Today I will mindfully connect my body and my soul.

Sharing in the Extraordinary Journey

~ Colleen Duggan-Cuomo, a Yogi

I am sharing an inspirational, exceptional-from-every-angle moment, experience from one of my students during a yoga class. This student had been practicing yoga with me for about six months. He used his imagination in a way that most of us as adults have "outgrown" or simply forgotten. I considered his beautiful, creative, imagination his superpower. This student also had the tendency of narrating every pose we did. One day during *Shavasana* (final relaxing pose of the class), he created imagery that I found brilliant. I typically guide students into relaxation through scanning their bodies for tension and systematically releasing it with visualization and breathwork. As his breath deepened, I could see and sense his body and mind relaxing, allowing his thoughts to dissolve and inviting in creative energy. Suddenly he said he was butter melting onto his mat made of toast.

The energy that he felt moving through his body was the sun melting him more and more deeply into the toast. What struck me most about this image was that from it, I knew he had an understanding of the effects that *prana* (energy) has on the body when we breathe in deeply. He had discovered what takes most of us years to figure out—that energy movement is real, tangible, and the desired result of yoga practice. This was amazing for me to experience, and I am honored to be the facilitator.

I Grow My Wisdom

Meditation

Meditation is used to rest the mind, body, and spirit. As you learn to rest your mind with intention and meditation, your ability to tune in to your higher faculties and wisdom becomes limitless. If that isn't enough of a reason, meditation also cultivates power through presence. It encompasses the energy of growth, creativity, nurturing, healing, joy, compassion, wisdom, emotional bonding, self-expression, empathy, and inner peace both individually and collectively. Meditation is not time-consuming. It is a planned activity when we open our minds, bodies, and spirits to connect with our inner beings through stillness and breath.

The Benefits of Meditation

- Calms the nervous system and decreases stress hormones.
- Circulates new energy and vitality into your life.
- Activates the energies of healing, growth, and peace, allowing the flow of connection between yourself and the universe.
- Allows you to slow down and accomplish what truly matters to you.

- Deepens your meaning of life and helps you to get more in sync with your inner being or spirit.
- Detoxes your mind of chatter and unwanted thoughts.
- Allows creative energy to surge through you to replenish, restore, and celebrate your life.
- Turns your attention inward and helps you listen to your inner wisdom and guidance.
- Provides an ideal time to release what doesn't serve your body.
- Teaches you to listen with your heart as you break free from your nonsensical mind chatter.
- Allows you to connect with your inner self, discovering the power to move through challenging times with more peace.
- Allows for inspiration and spontaneous impulse—defined as proceeding from natural feeling or tendency without external constraint, arising from a momentary impulse controlled and directed intentionally, and self-acting.

A dedication to the practice of meditation will produce a dramatic shift in your life. I use the word *dedication* because you must be patient and dedicated. It might not be easy right away, but dedicating eight to ten minutes a day of sacred space to nurture yourself will provide the long-term benefit of a peace and joy that is indescribable. This practice will help you set the perfect trajectory for the day by being present and giving you the power to see, hear, and think more clearly. Most importantly, it helps you make better decisions. Over time, we will all be more centered when faced with drama, obstacles, and crises.

For just a moment, reflect on all the outside stimulation in today's world to which you are subjected. Notice how often you are on autopilot with a cluttered mind. Is there a constant recycling of the past and worrying about the future, building stressors in your thinking? Ask yourself, "What kind of energy do I want influencing my life? What about my child's life?"

The American Academy of Pediatrics (AAP) states, "Our kids' brains are tired, and children of all ages really need opportunities where they can unplug to relax and focus. Meditation offers this break and helps kids function more efficiently and clearly." AAP encourages parents to share meditation with their children and teachers to incorporate mindfulness training into their lesson plans. Meditating is not rocket science, but it is dedication.

Meditation activity suggested times:

- Preschool: a few minutes per day.
- Grade school children: 3–10 minutes twice a day.
- Teens and adults: 5–30 minutes per day or more.

Allow yourself to get specific in how you will form this new habit, allowing for self-discovery, awareness, and consciousness to reconnect to your inner being and higher power. And once you have it, honor your own unique meditation practice. You can visualize roots extending from the soles of your feet, rooting deeply into the core of the earth. This is a common visualization in that it allows you to feel energetically secure and stable. Visualize yourself responding rather than reacting.

Just like brushing your teeth or with any new habit or routine, it works best to anchor it with an already well-established activity. For example, meditate each day after you brush your teeth or before you have your breakfast. Write it in your agenda and check it off when you complete it. This is a good way to establish a new habit.

Creating a safe, relaxing, feel-good energy space for yourself is key, but know this—you can't do it wrong! Thoughts will enter your mind. You will drift off. There is no question about that. Humans entertain sixty thousand to eighty thousand thoughts each day! When you drift away from the attention to your breath, that is okay. But when you realize you have, come back to it. Eventually, you will have fewer and fewer disruptions. You might get to five seconds without thoughts coming at you. Remember, progress over perfection!

Maybe your space will be on the floor with pillows. Maybe it will be in a comfy chair. Or maybe it will be sitting on a beanbag. Find a little nook where you can nestle in with a comfy blanket and pillow to support your back. The goal is to have a space that cultivates peace and quiet with positive energy, where you find yourself smiling more and more without any reason. This is a safe space to breathe in trust and exhale fear. You can meditate anywhere, but start in your home for now.

Items to use in creating a space that allows calming energy to flow:

- Weighted blanket.
- Cozy blanket, colorful pillows.
- Include nature into the space, such as seashells, feathers, or crystals.
- Cool rocks (put words like peace, positive, joy, quiet, happy, and love on each rock).
- Build a rock sculpture.
- Soothing photo(s).
- Candles and/or essential oils.
- Figurines.
- Art.
- Dream catcher (hang from window).
- Meditation cards/angel cards.
- Lava lamp, moon lights.
- A simple indoor, plug-in water fountain.
- Soft music, nature sounds, or whale and dolphin sounds.
- Guided meditation apps.
- Décor to inspire (for example, a globe to inspire travel).
- Plants.

Now that your beautiful, heartwarming space is set up, get comfortable. Set an intention for the day. Something that your heart desires. If you cannot think of any at first, go with what pops into your mind. And do not judge yourself—never judge yourself.

Tips to Guide Your Meditation

- Sit with your eyes closed or slightly open and focus on your breath and senses.
- Rest your hands on your belly (notice your belly rise and fall with each breath).
- Rest your hand on your heart (notice your chest rise and fall).
- Notice that when you breathe in, the air is cool.
- Notice that when you breathe out, the air is warmer.
- Notice any sounds in the room or outside.
- Notice any smells like something cooking, fresh cut grass, or flowers.

When you are quiet and paying attention to your senses, you naturally receive the messages you are meant to receive from the universe or higher power. It is practically impossible to receive the yumminess life has to offer when your mind is full of yesterday's junk. That junk is most likely blocking your energy to receive. Meditation is a time to release what doesn't serve your body.

Also know that some energy can be stuck from trauma on a cellular level in your tissues. Cells have memories, just like muscles. You have likely heard the phrase "muscle memory." This is similar. Often, interactions can poke at the traumatic memories and show up in our reactions, affecting our mood and energy. That is when you say to yourself, "Why did I overreact? Why did I say those things?" Yoga and meditation are healing modalities to help move energy that is stuck.

Yoga

Yoga is an intuitive energy practice. Energy permeates everything from our outer environment to our inner environment. You can't always control what is going on in the external world, but you absolutely have control of your inner environment. And you will be better equipped to manage your emotions and respond to the outside worldly concerns when you do so.

Implementing a yoga practice is instrumental in the exploration of finding your bliss. Yoga invites deep release of emotional and mental blockages that open your heart and mind for opportunities of expansion. It is more powerful than you could ever imagine. As you deepen your practice, you begin to feel and think lighter, creating more space, and allowing for self-discovery, awareness, and consciousness to reconnect to the innate power within you. It is in your power to create the most amazing day. As a dear friend of mine, Sherri Scaccia, yoga teacher, so beautifully said,

> Yoga poses are meant to 'create space' in our bodies, so we are open to accept the love and abundance that is our birthright. On our inhale we are 'expanding and opening,' and on our exhale we are 'releasing and emptying.' The deep dark spaces in our hips, chest, and shoulders hold baggage from our past, keeping us tight and bound to old memories, ideas, and beliefs. Yoga poses are meant to "open" these spaces and "empty" out the baggage. We do this with our breath. On the inhale, we "expand and open" those spaces. On the exhale, we "release and empty" that which no longer serves us. When we inhale our shoulders back and down, clasp our hands at our lower back and exhale our heart to the sky, we are "opening and emptying" the tight dark pocket between the shoulder and the chest, creating space, peace, and fluidity. Standing side bends, when done safely and intentionally, literally separate the ribs, opening the ribcage, creating more space for the breath to move freely about. And with a daily practice of hip openers (yogi squat, pigeon pose, crescent lunge) we are able to "open and release" this baggage, allowing for more flexibility and peace.

By digging into these pockets of emotions, and forgiving and letting go of whatever is there, we are creating space in our bodies, minds, hearts, souls, and spirits.

Mindfulness

Tanys Coughlan, Reiki Master & Celtic Shamanic High Priestess recommends the following when working with children on the autism spectrum:

> It is important to remember that they do not have the same attention span; some find it more difficult, while others can focus intently. Keep in mind that each child is different. You can start off by introducing them to coloring mandalas. They are circular and usually have a repeating geometric pattern. These are used in many cultures as a tool for meditation. They were historically done out of colored sand that would be placed in round repetitive patterns, and at the end, would be blown away. The reason for this was to remind the individual that nothing is permanent, and the only constant is change itself.
>
> You can find the mandala patterns now on the internet or books of them in your local bookstore. Coloring in the repetitive pattern provides a relaxing process of creativity. Children with special needs must have a creative outlet to release their pent-up creative energy. The action of coloring itself is a repetitive hand movement that allows the person coloring to relax into it. The pattern of the mandala is repetitive, so they can choose a color design and just repeat, which allows them to clear their mind as well. The children should be encouraged to use their creativity though, so if they choose to make everything different, that is okay too. It is important to note that the final product is not important. Rather, it is the process itself.
>
> Please allow your child to color as they wish and encourage them along the way if necessary. I have found it easier to provide colored pencils for this project, as the patterns can have small areas to get into. However, you are also able to find larger patterns if the child works better with crayons. I would provide colored pencils (or crayons), the mandalas, and a comfortable table at which to sit.

Then I would put on some soft music that contains *solfeggio* frequencies. These sounds act to create a change in the frequency of the brain and, in this case, a sense of relaxation. It has been found that a child can focus for longer periods with less body breaks than you would expect.

Next is the focused meditation. Keep the *solfeggio* frequencies going to maintain the relaxed brain waves. Breathing is very important for the body to deactivate the fight or flight response, so start by having them take some deep breaths and release. Then, ask them to close their eyes and picture their favorite place—one that makes them feel happy, safe, and secure. Ask them to think about what it looks like there, what it smells like, and what it feels like.

When you can create a connection between the senses and their safe and happy place, it can help them recreate the feelings they have when they are there and bring them into the present moment. This is an exercise that can help them relax at the end of the day, too. If you are doing it with one child instead of a group, have them answer the questions out loud, helping them maintain focus. You could also ask them to visualize colors representing the chakras of the energy system in order to activate the chakras. Then, end with three more deep breaths.

Cultivating a space that feels safe to share thoughts, giving time to form ideas, and to take stock of feelings is the key focus of mindfulness activities. You do not have to sit in one spot and be still to achieve a meditative state of mind. Basically, anything that they can drop into and focus attention on is a meditative state. This is building that mental muscle to be able to drop in and let go, creating calmness for the nervous system.

What makes it a mindful activity versus just an activity? Simply put, the parent is setting the intention that it is a mindful activity. The activity planned is instructed specifically to be mindful by getting them away from technology, TV, radio, and phone calls.

Let your child know this is going to be a mindful activity, a quiet activity to pay attention to what is going on around them by using their five senses. Look. Listen. Touch. Taste. Smell. Consistent mindful activities will help develop the mindful muscle, offering the nervous system some extended breaks!

I Ask My True Self

- *Where can I carve out fifteen minutes in my day to meditate?*
- *Do I need to get up earlier, meditate midday, or does evening work better?*
- *The next time I have a decision to make that I am unsure of, I will ask the question during my meditation and come closer to the right decision by paying attention to how this question makes me feel inside.*
- *Do I want to have more control of my inner environment—my body, mind, and spirit?*
- *Do I want to free my body and mind of the cobwebs of the past, releasing the negative energy attached that keeps me congested and feeling stuck?*

Aligning Thoughts with Actions

- Don't close the door to meditation and yoga for your children. These can be very helpful for them.
- Try one yoga pose at a time.
- Read a meditation card and talk about it with your child.
- Incorporate mindfulness activities into your routine and your child's:
    - Drawing
    - Coloring
    - Cooking
    - Building a rock sculpture
    - Collecting seashells at the beach
    - Blueberry picking
    - Walking through the woods, touching trees
    - Finding and making a gratitude rock

- Ask these questions after the mindful activity with open-ended, engaging communication:
    - How is your body feeling right now?
    - How do your feet feel on the ground?
    - How do your clothes feel?
    - Do you taste anything in your mouth, even if you're not eating? Cultivating a mindful activity rather than an ordinary activity makes a huge difference.
- Practice the Paradise Is Closer than You Think Meditation Game
    - Set a time to meditate (maybe three minutes to start).
    - Each time you drift away and start thinking about other things, point one finger up.
    - Measure your mental muscle focus. Over time, you will see fewer fingers up in the game.
- Practice the Razor's Edge Focus Drill
    - Place a lit candle or another object about fifteen feet away.
    - Sit in a chair and keep your eyes focused on the object or even a dot on the wall.
    - Have a timer or a watch.
    - Stare at the candle or dot on the wall as long as you can. When you blink, record the time. Strive to focus a couple of seconds longer each time and you will see your focus time improve.

Colleen Duggan-Cuomo, Yoga teacher recommends:

Use a deck of "yoga cards" to map out sequences of postures. This allows students to practice at their own pace and to explore, and be creative with, different poses. Students can interpret each pose in a way that works with their special abilities. Some students have responded well to repeating sequences of three or four poses. At home, keeping a yoga mat out and about is a great way to invite your child to explore yoga.

Reflections of the Soul . . .

Happiness is an inside job.

~ William Arthur Ward

Reflections of the Soul . . .

If you change the way you look at things, the things you look at change.

~ Wayne Dyer

Chapter 9

Lessons from the Moon

Capturing the Energy of the Sky

Positive Affirmation

Today I will use the energy around me to build me up.

Sharing in the Extraordinary Journey

~ Nicole Donovan, Mother and Author of *A Life Suspended: A Mother and Son's Story of Autism, Extinction Bursts, and Living a Resilient Life*

Jack was older when I began practicing rituals, and he resisted them, which was fine. I didn't push. We had some good conversations about spirituality sprinkled in over the years, but only when they organically presented themselves. Over about five years though, he had seen me do my spiritual practices—clearing the house with sage, meditating, reading cards, and putting out crystals and jars of water under the full moon. Jack often points out to me when the moon is full. He seems to like that I chase the moon and take photos.

What I have learned raising older kids is that they are always watching. At some point during the teen years, they stop "listening" to parental guidance, but their eyes are still taking it all in.

Jack's greatest love is history—ancient Egypt, in particular. He collects figurines, art, and items that are Egyptian themed. A few years ago, I noticed he arranged them on a tray. He made an altar of sorts. When I pointed it out, he laughed, shrugged his shoulders, and said "Well, I guess I did!" Most recently, while on vacation, Jack went antiquing. He found a framed Egyptian papyrus of King Tut and bought it with his own money. Later, he found a pendulum at another shop and bought that because he has "always been curious about them." These purchases were all on his own, with no input from me.

Jack, like most kids in the tween or teen years, may not be interested in being taught something new, but if we are doing these practices because we find them spiritually and emotionally filling, we are creating opportunities for our kids to watch, ask questions, and create their own beliefs and practices. What we do, what we say, and our intentions all ripple out to our children, to our homes, and to our environments.

~ Cynthia Kahler, Single Working Mom

I find myself having the desire to explore my spirituality and doing inner work to let go and move forward, including connecting with nature more, increasing gratitude, thinking more positively, striving to be the best version of myself, and allowing my son to do the same. I took a chance and asked Jack to participate in a full moon ritual. I explained that we would both write things down that were bothering us on a piece of paper—things on our mind that we wanted to be rid of. I explained that we would go outside on the eve of the full moon and under the energy of the moon and stars, we would release those thoughts to the universe by throwing the paper in the firepit and watching it burn. Surprisingly, Jack said yes. We both prepared for the full moon by writing down everything that was bothering us and our minds that we wanted to get rid of.

On the night of the full moon, we built a fire in our firepit, and we thought about what we wrote down on the paper and threw it into the firepit and watched it burn.

When asked, Jack shared his experience of the full moon ritual:

> *On a small piece of paper, we wrote down everything that was bothering us and then we threw the papers into the fire we lit, and it symbolized those problems going away.*

I asked Jack how the full moon ritual made him feel.

> *It made me feel good.*

I asked Jack, "Have you ever done this kind of thing before in any of your therapy over all the years?"

> *No.*

I asked Jack, "Did you find this helpful? Would you do it again?"

> *Yes.*

I Grow My Wisdom

New Moon

The new moon occurs on a monthly cycle. It is a time to gather in the magnificence and bountiful energy of the new moon, stars, and universe. Take this opportunity to connect with the infinite universe, recognizing its abundance and limitlessness. Picture yourself sitting on another planet looking down at Earth. What do you see now? How do you feel? With your bird's eye view, you can now see with more clarity the uniqueness of each snowflake, grain of sand, raindrop, rock, mountain, river, tree, and flower. Think of other things you see from your view sitting above the world.

The new moon is a time to set intentions, create goals, and begin new projects, planting the seeds of your heartfelt desires. Without a doubt, this is a beautiful, empowering, purposeful practice to embrace. Picture in your mind a treasure box. What does your treasure box look like? Inside are your wants, desires, gifts, and maybe something you have always wanted to do or be but never thought it was possible. What do you wish to accomplish? What rockets of desire do you want to ignite and lift off to the new moon, radiating energy and building momentum?

The new moon's energy helps fuel your rockets of desire. Connecting with a higher power always leaves you feeling calm, serene, hopeful, and empowered, with knowledge that you are never alone, you are guided, you are safe, and you are free—free to move and free to edit your story as you write it. Visualize in your mind a blank white canvas on an art easel and see your list magically appearing in script, including questions to which you are looking for answers.

Everyone should write their goals, heart's desires, projects, and new habits on a piece of paper. Writing it out and vocalizing with expression gives more energy to your wants. It is your practice, so what feels right to you is right.

Benefits:

- Family engagement is a magnificent way to link connections with your true self, your family, and the universe.
- This is a wonderful opportunity to hear what your child wants or needs in a form of expression that is never judged.
- This is a time to share, discover, and support each other.

- Making a habit of asking permission is a fantastic way to show respect for your child's thoughts and feelings.
- Asking permission builds confidence and self-esteem.
- This is yet another chance to reprogram your mind to think in a certain way, allowing creative energy thinking.

Full Moon

The full moon is also monthly. Like the new moon, it creates an opportunity for a new tradition for yourself and your family, creating connectivity and opening the heart. This is an opportunity to:

- develop self-trust,
- step into bravery,
- create a deepening practice to shed the formalities, and
- get to know who you really are.

This is a time to sit under the moon and meditate for a few minutes, release what doesn't serve you, and offer gratitude for the beauty of your life and your child. You are resolving the things you want to release. Start with sharing something you admire about each person or something for which you are grateful, inviting a feel-good, safe space for all. This allows positive energy to flow and more freedom to release and let go of fear, anger, headaches, stomachaches, or guilt. This gives you the space to discover what may be weighing your child down.

I Ask My True Self

- *What do I want guidance with—healing, a vision, a habit, a goal, or peace?*
- *How can I live so that my inner beliefs and outer actions are in alignment?*
- *How can I resonate better with my inner beliefs and incorporate habits that feel good to me?*

- *When is the next new moon? Full moon?*
- *Will I engage in these practices and help my child do so?*

Aligning Thoughts with Actions

Ideas for new moon rituals:

- Write the words "Rockets of Desire" and "Release What Does Not Serve Me" on the dates of the new moon and full moon, respectively, on your calendar.
- On the eve of the new moon, gather in the yard, on the porch or deck, or even on the beach.
- Light a candle or have an outdoor fire. Light is a symbol of awareness.
- Personalize the space with a rock, crystal, figurine, essential oil, or a photo that brings comfort.
- Each person says out loud (or to themselves) what they wrote on their paper.
- Visualizing on the screen of your mind, writing it out, and vocalizing with expression— all create energy. Whether you chose one or all is up to you.
- Your personal ritual will expand naturally as you continue monthly.
- Ask the universe for guidance or help. Ask the questions. Ask to place people and events in your life on your path to help you achieve your heart's desires.
- Offer gratitude—give thanks for this guidance.
- Keep your written goals and wants displayed in a place you will see often. You can put them in a frame or tape a list to the mirror in the bathroom. You can also put it in a protective sheet, keep it by your bed, or put it under your pillow.
- If your child does not want to participate, you can still do this and allow your child to watch.
- Continue monthly.

- Consider that the Farmers' Almanac includes moon phases and dates, gardening, and long-term forecasts.

Ideas for the full moon ritual:

The preparation is similar, and you can follow the same steps to the new moon ritual except for these few differences:

- Each person writes down what they want to release.
- If it feels right, share.
- Each person throws the paper into the fire after reading it, symbolically letting go. It feels good. Your vibration will be raised with this process.
- Ask for guidance and help in assisting your release.

Reflections of the New Moon . . .

Whatever you fear most has no power. It is your fear that has the power.

~ Oprah Winfrey

Reflections of the Full Moon . . .

There is no Wi-Fi in the forest, but I promise you will find a better connection.

~ Ralph Smart

Chapter 10

Worthy Goals

Set Them, Work toward Them,
Achieve Them!

Positive Affirmation

Today I will set a new goal, work toward one, or achieve one.
I may do all three!

Sharing in the Extraordinary Journey

~ Cynthia Kahler, Single Working Mom

My son, Jack, 19, set a goal that he wanted to go to college. Jack has always struggled with his autism diagnosis. He wanted to be like a "typical" kid—one who goes to college, gets a job, and one day has a family. All of these were overwhelming to him since he struggles with anxiety about new things. Knowing Jack as I do, I knew he could accomplish his desires and goals; he just needed to build the confidence that he deserved it.

I felt that if Jack had the opportunity to be in a college setting, it would help him be reassured that he could break through his fears and move forward with his goals. I went about looking for a program for kids on the autism spectrum that would provide a supportive college experience. We explored colleges like Dean and Mitchell that have wonderful full time college programs for kids who need support. Still, feelings of fear of success were lingering when we came upon the College Internship Program. Its objective is to provide kids with a taste of independence and college living. This sounded like a great first step toward his set goal of attending college. Jack was open to it and made the decision to attend. He was very afraid of leaving home and me. His famous line is *I just don't know what to expect.* I replied that the unknown can be scary, but exciting too.

Jack's intention all along was to stay for the full ten days the program offered. He faced his fears of being away from home to gain a better understanding of the college experience and explore his goal of going one day. Jack set a very worthy goal—one that stretched him, scared him, and excited him at the same time.

When the day came for Jack to go, he was very anxious, as was I. I asked him if I told him he didn't have to go, would he want to go back home. He adamantly said, "No way! I am doing this!" We got to the dorm and got him settled. He was crying as I left him. I think I cried for almost half the ride home, thinking to myself *how did I just leave my autistic kid in the middle of nowhere?*

I texted Jack Monday and Wednesday that week but never received a response. I could track his cell phone, so thankfully, I knew he was still there. As part of the curriculum, they were supposed to call home Wednesday night. I anxiously awaited his call and was very concerned I didn't hear from him. I didn't know if that meant he was doing great or awful. I found out later that Jack had called his dad on Monday night and told him to tell me not to call him or text him—he was missing me and home very much and he said it was going to be too hard to hear my voice. He told his dad to tell me he missed me, loved me, and that he was doing alright.

I really wanted to hear his voice, but I thought, *wow—how intuitive of him to not only recognize his feelings, but also to come up with a plan and course of action to manage his emotions.* I thought this was brilliant. He knew exactly what he needed to do and how to manage his emotions to stay at camp and achieve his goal of attending until the end. He was committed to working through his fears and managing his emotions recognizing every day it was a little bit easier. I was so proud!

Day five was a milestone and a huge sense of accomplishment for Jack—he was tear free. He was not as homesick and was able to take in more of the college experience. He finally called Thursday afternoon. He was doing okay and was settling in. He actually sounded a LOT better than I had expected. He said he was getting used to the place. I was so excited for him to be doing this!

The last day came, and Jack had done it! He achieved a worthy goal. He felt a sense of accomplishment that he actually lived away from home for almost two weeks! I was beyond proud of him!

~ Patrice Headd, M.Ed., Special Education, Pre-School Teacher

Most of us can remember a joyful nursery rhyme we learned as a child. Why does that memory stick? The power of repetition and using all our senses when we learn multiplies the neural brain connection activity that happens during the learning process.

As a preschool teacher in special education, while planning a nursery rhyme lesson, I visualize my students becoming fully engaged, joyfully singing the verses, and using their bodies to move and act out the story over and over again throughout the year. Children love repetition and gain in all areas of learning—academic, physical, social, and emotional— while using this approach, and their confidence soars. Every day in my classroom, I see firsthand how this tool engages my little learners physically and cognitively, which makes learning fun, effective and meaningful. Using our senses and the tool of the repetition while learning helps build a strong brain and develop a love of learning that will last a lifetime. This is a great tool to use when setting goals.

I Grow My Wisdom

When setting a worthy goal, it should be something that you don't already know how to do. For example, "My goal is to do laundry today" is not a worthy goal. You already know how to do laundry. Your goal should be something special, something important to you, and you must really want it. Once you choose a goal, it should excite you and scare you at the same time, especially if the goal is a "stretch" for you, propelling you to grow and get out of your comfort zone.

Goal setters do not put limits on what they can accomplish. Instead, they get out of their comfort zone and acknowledge that it is there where you learn and grow. As you pursue your goals, give yourself the space and permission to have downs, along with your ups. There will be setbacks, but true growth only occurs during those times. Allowing yourself the time and space to feel what you need to feel with these experiences and then picking yourself back up is allowing for grace in your life. This also cultivates a message of resilience and never giving up on your heart's desires. We must learn to embrace the struggle and love the challenge, understanding that we only see light through dark. And that it's at these times of discomfort and pain when we are growing into the most brilliant, best version of ourselves.

The journey of reaching your goal improves the overall happiness in your life. In your comfort zone, you know what to expect, and it is something you are familiar with, so you stay there, gaining no personal growth. Sometimes people stay in that safe/comfort zone their whole lives, and that is okay too. Most people don't even realize this. The real purpose of a goal is to learn and achieve new things in life as you work toward it.

You must fully expect to achieve your goal. You are sincerely interested in improving the quality of your life. In fact, you are not only interested, but committed. So, stop second guessing yourself!

- Elevate your ambitions and learn from the brightest minds.
- Connect with peers from around the world, and build relationships that offer support and opportunity through networking groups, support groups, meet-ups, and book clubs.
- Be inspired by the energy of others, events, workshops, and personal development podcasts that will ignite your action plans and renewed passion to carry on with your vision.
- Get ahead of the crowd by arming yourself with the most up-to-date research and knowledge. Explore current topics and trends related to your goals.
- Seek out and take action on opportunities and solutions to challenges. Act on opportunities that may arise unexpectedly.

Repetition in Achieving Goals

Repetition is the Universal Law of Learning. A message heard over and over is much more likely to stay in your mind. Words and thoughts that are repeated get stronger through repetition and then sink into the subconscious mind and affect behavior, actions, and reactions. Most people already do this subconsciously. But when you do this with conscious intention, you will emit an electric surge of energy that will accelerate the process. This is especially powerful in achieving your goals.

For example, when studying, reading, or listening to a chapter or lesson, sometimes you might read the words while your thoughts drift off elsewhere. Then you come back to the book realizing you are lost—you missed something and need to reread or rewind it. This happens all the time. Your thoughts are a distraction to the task at hand. Programming the mind to be more focused has everything to do with repetition.

Read it, see it (imagine it), then read it out loud, and allow your emotions to get involved in what you are studying, so you can absorb it. The power of repetition is a key strategy in behavior change. Work toward your goals and desires by reprogramming the mind with repetition. Reading and practicing these tools repeatedly are the keys that unlock the freedom within.

On the opposite side, when someone tells a lie and they repeat it over and over, to the point where they become emotionally attached to the lie, they are also reprogramming their minds. Demonstrating the above, what you tell yourself repeatedly becomes your reality. They tell their lie for so long, with so much feeling, conviction, and certainty that they actually believe it. It becomes their reality. Their true version. The same holds true in believing in yourself to accomplish your goal. It takes repetition of the reality you desire, the change you want to accomplish!

Information combined with an emotion becomes a long-term memory. This helps explain why when you hear a song from childhood, you remember the emotion you felt at that time. It could also be a fragrance or food that stimulates the memory and brings you back decades. Elevating the state of mind to something that you or your child enjoys prior to the learning of something new could be as simple as talking about a video game they like or something else in which they have an interest, elevating the state of mind to receive new information. Sharing in a playful, imaginative visualization is a great way to help with your transition to new things. We can also heighten our state of mind through movement. Thoughts that you express with feeling and emotion give energy to your words and can shape your life.

When you declare conscious intention of a goal or your happy place, and involve all your senses, it propels you forward and begins to take on a whole new form. The repetition and visualization of your happy place and your goals sharpens the senses, promotes intuition, and helps you to be practical, centered, and grounded. Conscious commitment of repeatedly writing your goal paired with visualization (like watching a motion picture on the screen of your mind), along with stating your intention out loud with feeling, gives vibration to your energy. Listening to your voice builds trust in yourself. You become what you think about.

Repetition is necessary when changing your beliefs, habits, and mindset. Through repetition, using all of your senses, you will connect to what is important to you and be better equipped to achieve your goals.

See it. Write it. Say it. Feel it. Smell it. Repeat. I am reprogramming my mind to think in a certain way.

I Ask My True Self

- *What does my heart truly desire?*
- *Make your list. If nothing comes right away, it is okay. Keep asking and let your mind wander through possibilities. Make time to keep thinking about it.*
- *What have I always dreamed of?*
- *What puts a smile on my face?*
- *What would make me wake up in the morning eager to start my day?*
- *Why is the power of repetition so crucial to make change?*
- *What change do I desire?*
- *How can I apply the power of repetition tool to change a belief or habit to move me toward a better version of me?*

Aligning Thoughts with Actions

- Declare your intention to be a committed goal setter.
- Remember, there is a difference between being interested in creating the life you want and being committed to creating the life you want. When you are interested, you do what is convenient. When you are committed, you do whatever it takes.
- Accept only results, not excuses.

- Make a list of thirty things you would really want, have, or change, if money were not a limitation. If you could have anything your heart desires, what would it be? Do not hold back. Fantasize and write your list.
- Create three categories: personal goals, health goals, and professional/career goals.
- List ten things under each category, then prioritize 1–10.
- Take the number one goal from each category.
- Now you have three worthy goals!
- Choose the one you want to accomplish the most. Don't analyze it. Which one will make you feel the best and give you the most excitement?
- Declare that you are worthy of the good you desire.
- Make a Goal Card.
  - Start with, "I am so happy and grateful now that . . ."
  - Write your goal on a colored index card, including a goal achievement date. (This is an estimation, but make sure you include it.)
  - The purpose of the goal card is to be a constant reminder of your goal.
  - Carry your goal card in your pocket or pocketbook, or keep it in a place where you see it throughout the day.
- Create a vision board of your goal. Make a habit of looking at it while brushing your teeth every day and night.
- Make a habit of spending five minutes fantasizing about your goal daily.
- Visualize people congratulating you on meeting your goal.
- Write your goal and describe it in your journal in detail.
- Share your goal with others. This is so important. The more you talk about it, with passion and certainty, the more energy is infused into

your goal, allowing you to open yourself to inspiration and action toward it.

- Do one thing that moves you closer to your goal every day. Write that one thing down before you go to bed at night.
- Record the written goal in your own voice using the video feature on a cell phone (or record your voice only, if desired). Listen to this recording before bed, while you are in the car, on a walk, or while you're cooking dinner.

Reflections of Goals . . .

Your past does not predict your future. Trust your gut, not your fears and pursue your goals.

~ Neil Wood

Reflections of Goals . . .

All progress takes place outside the comfort zone.

~ Michael John Bobak

Chapter 11

Simple Solutions

Make Decisions and Focus on the Results

Positive Affirmation

Today I will make the best decisions for my child and me.

Sharing in the Extraordinary Journey

~ Lisa Drennan, MERGE Diverse Abilities Inclusion Consulting; Let's Get to Success Approach

This principle of inclusion is about having a change in perspective or mindset that helps us to be more solution- and results-focused. It is rooted in the concept that when approached with a challenging predicament, we seek to have a "Let's Get to Success" attitude.

Let's say your child has asked to sign up for a traditional camp instead of the special needs one she has always attended because her friend from school is going there this summer. Your first thoughts may be to start listing the "what ifs," and the reasons why "this won't work." You start to focus on all that could go wrong: *What if they don't know how to deal with her if she has a meltdown? What if kids make fun of her speech impairment? What if she can't keep up with the instruction of the activities?*

Instead, this principle of inclusion would suggest that when approached with a predicament like this, you take a deep breath in, pause for a moment, and say to yourself, *How can we make this work?* Then tap into all your resources to explore how to make it happen. In this case, it might be talking to the camp director, asking other members of her support network (and your daughter) for suggestions and solutions on how to make this a success, and preparing her by creating a social story and touring the camp ahead of time.

This simple mindset shift sets an example for your child that when you set your mind to something and work together with all involved, you can set and accomplish your goals and make your dreams a reality.

I Grow My Wisdom

You have always had the will, and now you have the way. How you respond and what you view as an obstacle or problem determines how you move through finding the solutions with ease and confidence. When you take a bird's eye view, you can see the situation from every angle. Soaring above the earth expands your view of the situation, allowing you to see more options and opportunities. As you learn to look for the exceptional from every angle, you will be led to more solutions than you ever imagined.

First, obsessing over your wounds, recycling the old should have/could have scenarios, and playing the blame game prevent you from moving forward. Think of it this way—it is usually not the problem that causes your suffering, it is your incessant thinking about the problem. A mind cluttered with fear, doubt, and blame makes it next to impossible to have clarity to find a possible solution. You are in a tunnel vision that keeps diminishing and restricts you mentally, physically, and spiritually.

The truth is that there are many different solutions right at your front door. However, your tunnel vision or perception of the problem becomes too narrow. The door is not only closed, but behind the door, stuff is piled so high that you can't see anything other than clutter, creating panic, anxiety, and reactiveness.

All too often, we rely on others to find the solution, because we do not trust ourselves to decide what is best for us. So, we find ourselves asking others what we should do or what the smartest thing for us to do is. The people we are asking may or may not have the best intentions for us, and they are offering advice based on their own past experiences. Subconsciously, we ignore our intuition because we think others know better or we are just not aware that we have the answers within us already.

When you look at obstacles as opportunities, you allow for understanding that the challenge happened for a reason—that something good will come out of it. Even if we can't see it in the moment, just knowing it will show up at some point is enough. Taking this attitude helps you automatically feel better, letting go of resistance and frustration with the situation. You are now energetically in the flow of inspiration, and you will be amazed by how many solutions drop into your mind when you practice thinking and acting in this way.

As you continue your journey to self-discovery, awareness, and consciousness, you begin to trust and rely on yourself for the answers you are seeking. As you get better at listening to your intuition and your gut feelings, rather than what your mind is chattering about, you become more decisive. Gut feelings always come from the heart, instinctively. You just need to tap back into that space. This is how I interpret the saying, *You have everything you need inside of you.*

Your decision to make a shift by thinking in a certain way guides you to learn more through a willingness to see love in all things and circumstances. When I use the word "shift," I refer to a desired change in your thinking, perception, and being. The desire alone to release resistance, let go of your pain, and trust your healing journey is extremely powerful. The transformation of your being brings a richness, an aliveness with inspiration of purpose. You will see that any problem can be looked upon as an opportunity to be more, do more, and give more. In this mindset, you will be soaking up and pouring out more happiness!

When you look for the good in a problem or circumstance, it allows the flow of more positive thinking to solve the problem, because you let go of the resistance or frustration attached to it. Take the bird's eye view, looking for the exceptional from every angle.

Simplify Decision Making

People who are good decision makers have developed their intuition and allow their feelings and inner selves to guide them. Learn to listen to your heart rather than the random chatter in your mind. Refer to your tools of conscious breathing and body scans to clear your mind before making any important decisions.

Ask yourself, how does this decision make my heart feel? If it is a *hell yeah*, then it's probably a great decision. If you're excited and a little scared, that is usually a good sign. If you are going back and forth, it's probably not a good decision at this moment. Meditation and asking questions will help to clarify your position. If you are feeling anxious and nervous, the timing is likely not right at this moment and you should hold off on the yes decision. If you are not ready to commit to a decision, and are feeling off, go with your gut. If you are saying the words, "I should," then definitely hold off, as it is probably not the right decision, at least right now.

Be aware of the word *should*. Have you ever been asked to decide something, and your thoughts are telling you that you should do it? Pause before you make any final decision, as this is a red flag. When you feel you *should* decide a certain way, your decision is based on other people's beliefs that have been impressed upon you. This is most likely conditioning from childhood. Whether it was your upbringing or whether your opinion has been influenced by someone else doesn't matter at this point, it is plain and simple that you don't really want to do it.

When it comes to your children, try to allow them to make their own decisions. Learning how to make decisions brings order and clarity to the mind and builds confidence. Teaching your child to pay attention to how their body feels when asked to do something will develop their intuition and simplify decision making for them. Ask this important question when deciding: Does this decision, circumstance, or person make you feel more in the element of creating or disintegrating? The element of creation is moving forward . . . striving and thriving. The element of disintegrating is moving backward. Once you stop learning about yourself and exploring life, you are either staying stuck where you are or moving backward, disintegrating.

Increase your awareness of your feelings, rather than navigating the confusion in your mind when making decisions. The answer is so much more obvious when you go within for the answer, connecting with your inner being and allowing the energy you feel to support your decision. Sometimes, the answer jumps out at you. Sometimes, you need to get still, pause, and allow your feelings to align with your thoughts around the situation, circumstance, person, or question. By making this a routine or habit, the answer becomes clear. As you strengthen this skill, making decisions gets easier, as does life in general.

Finally, as you make decisions and find solutions, trust the timing in your life. Sometimes, we still do not make the best decisions, and it's important to know that it is okay and part of the learning process in developing who we are. Instead of looking at it as poor decision making, look at it as a stepping-stone and you will feel better about the situation. It is our life experiences—the good, the bad, and the ugly—that shape us into the person we are. Do not beat yourself up over it. Accept it and move forward.

I Ask My True Self

- *Is there a problem or obstacle I am currently faced with?*
- *Can I look deeper and find an opportunity or find something good that could come out of the obstacle?*
- *What do I need to feel safe right now?*
- *What do I need to feel seen right now?*
- *What do I need to feel soothed right now?*
- *What do I need to feel secure right now?*

Aligning Thoughts with Actions

Behavior Change Specialist Tips:

- Acknowledge the problem.
- Clearly state the obstacle and write it down.
- Brainstorm all the possible outcomes.
- Write down your desired outcome.
- Put a big "X" over the outcomes you know you don't want.
- Allow creative energy thinking and ask yourself, "How can I find something good in this situation?"
- Know there is an opportunity in this obstacle. You just need to find one positive thing that can or will come out of it.
- Your new view of problems or obstacles is that they are opportunities for expansion and personal growth.

Tips to help you become a decisive decision maker:

- Trust and pay attention to your feelings—let them guide you to your decision.
- Be aware of the word "should."
- Trust there is an omniscient "knowing" that even if it is not the best decision, it is a stepping-stone to becoming a better decision maker.

- Give yourself permission to make poor decisions, and expect it will happen at times.
- When you make a poor decision, protect your energy.
- Most importantly, follow your heart's desire. If it is a *Hell Yeah!* do it and don't let anything stop you. You are worthy.
- Recognize when your paradigm is holding you back. Then plow through it.
- Know with certainty that you are worthy and deserve to invest in yourself. Choose to ignite that inner spark and let it fire you up!
- Choose to be alive in your life, not just to live.

Reflections of Solutions . . .

It is not what you do for your children, but what you have taught them to do for themselves, that will make them successful human beings.

~ Ann Landers

Reflections of Solutions . . .

You can't lead anyone else further than you have gone yourself.

~ Gene Mauch

Author's Note

Sharing a Piece of My Heart

It is my sincere hope that the lessons and practices in this book help parents of children on the autism spectrum move obstacles out of their way. Maybe they will all resonate with you, or maybe certain ones will more than others. That's okay; give yourself grace, and take what you can, where you can. Truly understanding the power you have within your mind will help your child understand their own. Remember, you are their superhero, so use these practices as your life raft, and power through.

I want to leave you with a personal story of a true breathing meditation visualization I experienced on a day of complete and utter hopelessness. My son came to me telling me that he was wishing for disease to take him. He explained he would never commit suicide because he didn't want to do that to me. I was, of course, devastated. Days later, I went to the beach. I now realize that I was guided to the beach on a cold winter's day for a bigger reason than I could have imagined. This day served me beyond my imagination.

I was walking along the beach and then sat quietly, bundled up with my hat and mittens in desperation. I was facing the ocean but looking up at the sky. I knew I needed help. As I searched the sky for answers, I saw clouds that formed a whimsical angel's wing. I was so amazed that I grabbed my phone and took a picture. I sat trying to immerse myself in the sound of the ocean waves and to stop the chattering thoughts of the dark places my mind was taking me. I visualized myself on a life raft and created in my imagination the most beautiful, incredible happy place.

As I came out of my meditative state, I found myself asking for help out loud. I even drew a heart in the sand with the word HELP, adding my son's name and his date of birth. Again, I found some quiet space in between my thoughts to listen. Unexpectedly, I felt my heart open, and I received a spontaneous impulse, like someone was tapping me on the shoulder, saying, "You are never alone, you can do this." In that moment, my eyes teared up. I was not sure, but I felt they were tears of joy. I surrendered. I surrendered to the invisible, choosing faith over fear to be the light penetrating directly into my son's heart. I visualized him smiling and healing, and sent him unconditional love, compassion, and forgiveness. I felt a wave of relief. I was able to dig deep, gathering all the strength within to give to him.

Clear as day, I saw that I was exactly where I was supposed to be that day. I now honor and give thanks to that day. I see this as one of the best days of my life, as this place of hopelessness brought me to a place of surrender and the experience of a higher power guiding me. Only when I became the best version of myself could I be the light and hold sacred space for my son to heal with the understanding he needed. And he did heal. But I could not control it. I could not fix it. I accepted that and chose faith over fear.

My hope is that you will do the same.

Knowledge Is Power . . .
Terms to Master

Positive Affirmation: Today I am a knowledge seeker!

Autonomy: The quality of being self-governing.

Cognitive Empathy: Having an understanding about how another thinks and feels.

Defense: To keep someone or something safe.

Disengagement: Marked by poor eye contact; distracted behaviors, such as looking at the television, computer, phone, or text messaging, or not participating in conversation.

Emotional Empathy: Feeling another's emotions along with the person.

Emotional Intelligence (EQ): The ability to recognize, interpret, and manage emotions positively in oneself and in others.

Empathetic Concern: An emotional response based on compassion and concern.

Internal Motivation: Motivation to accomplish a goal that comes from within.

Managing Discord: Recognizing the discord or conflict, regardless of the type, and responding to it immediately.

Positive Psychology: The study of the strengths that enable individuals, families, and communities to thrive. This belief is founded on the idea that people want to lead meaningful and fulfilling lives, to cultivate what is best within themselves, and to enhance their experiences of love, work, and play.

Rapport: A relationship marked by mutual trust and understanding.

Reflective Listening: A special type of listening in which a person is respectfully paying attention to what someone else is saying and acknowledges it to that person.

Self-Awareness: Ability to identify one's own emotions, behaviors, traits, and feelings.

Self-Efficacy: A belief in one's own capacity to accomplish tasks or goals.

Self-Management: Also called self-control. The ability to use emotions and behaviors effectively in different situations.

Social Awareness: The ability to see various perspectives and empathize with others, including those with diverse backgrounds.

Squaring Off: A signal that one feels an adversarial relationship with the other person. Typically squaring off statements come in the form of "you" statements (e.g., "You don't understand," "You don't know what it's like to be me," "You are wrong.")

Contributors to *Sharing in the Extraordinary Journey*

Tanys Coughlan

Reiki Master and Intuitive Energy and Crystal Healer, International Teacher and Speaker, Founder of the Twillow Lifestyle Community and the Twillow Lifestyle Academy

The Twillow Lifestyle Community is helping people live up to their highest potential by providing training, healing, and coaching in a compassionate and safe environment that supports their spiritual, emotional, and physical needs.

www.twillowlifestyle.ca

Coleen Duggan ~ Cuomo, Yogi: Founder and Owner of Breathing Lotus Living Arts, Kingston, Ma

Nicole Dauz
Self-care Coach, Speaker, and Author

Reclaim your happiness. Nicole's mission is to help every parent regain control of their lives, so they can find the pieces of themselves they lost when they became caregivers.

www.nicoledauz.com

Lisa Drennan
Founder, MERGE Diverse Abilities Inclusion Consulting

Building stronger communities by providing expert guidance to recreational organizations on inclusion of persons with diverse abilities.
www.mergeconsulting.org

Nicole Hendrick Donovan
Author, Reflective Storyteller, and Guide

Nicole's memoir *A Life Suspended: A Mother and Son's Story of Autism, Extinction Bursts, and Living a Resilient Life* brings the reader into the home and heart of a family in crisis. It is a story about a mother's unwavering love and finding hope in ordinary things. Nicole is the owner of Rose Ray Healing Arts, which houses a line of self-care products, crystal bowl sound healing, Reiki energy sessions, coaching, meditation classes, and workshops.

www.nhdwrites.com

Patrice Headd M.Ed., Special Education, Pre-School Teacher

Cynthia Kahler ~ Mom of Jack, single working mom

Heidi Rome

Autism Mom, Author, Speaker, Educator, Severe Autism Discourse Changer, and Question Asker. Her memoir *You Just Have to Love Me* shares the wisdom of her nonspeaking son Ethan, reminding us that our humanity shows that our only job is to love and accept each other. There is no fixing because no one is broken—not the autistic child, and not the mom. Just breathe. Just love.

www.heidirome.com

Sherri Scaccia yoga teacher offers a passage on creating space in the body through yoga poses, pg. 101

Richard Schreiber
Founder, NYC Autism Community Group

Promoting and championing alternative and working solutions for autistic people young and old, as well as their support networks and families. Providing alternatives to mainstream and pharmaceutical options.

www.nycautismcommunity.org

Elizabeth Joy Shaffer
OTD, OTR/L, ODT/L Founder of Therapeutic Innovations International, Pediatric Occupational Therapist

Mom, Educator, Speaker, and Neurodivergent Individual

Elizabeth helps parents and children worldwide by providing holistic tools and techniques to self-regulate through life's stresses, mindfully work through difficult moments, and experience more joy in everyday life.
www.therapyintl.com

Adam Szecowka
Autism Specialist, Global Intuitive Energy Healer, and Author

Identifying and successfully addressing the "true" root causes of the individual's challenges deep down from even beyond the cellular levels and taking environmental factors into consideration provides you with the keys to both the short- and long-term positive changes the whole family can experience. All services are 100 percent custom designed to meet the unique requirements of each individual.

www.alchemyspectrum.com

Resources

Autism Eats

Provides autism-friendly, non-judgmental restaurant dining events. Families can socialize, connect, and have fun with others who share similar joys and challenges.

www.autismeats.org

The Catastrophic Illness in Children Relief Fund (CICRF)

A little-known federal program that assists families who are spending more than 10% of their annual income on unreimbursed medical expenses for their disabled minor children, including costs for therapeutic services associated with an autism diagnosis. Reach out to the CICRF administrative agency in your state to find out if you are eligible and how to apply.

Positive Affirmations for Parents

https://unlimitedplay.org/10-encouraging-affirmations-for-parents/*Positive Affirmations for Kids: 101 Positive Affirmation*

Hearts to be Heard: Giving a Voice to Creativity

Their mission is to give a voice to heartfelt creativity for those who otherwise would not be heard. A voice will be given to the creativity that lies within the hearts of our children living with diverse challenges. Children who have the opportunity to have their hearts heard will have the freedom to create beautiful works of art and music.

www.heartstobeheard.com

Insight Timer ~ Free App

Guided meditations. Helps calm the mind, reduce anxiety, manage stress, sleep, and improve happiness.

Calm ~ Free App

Guided meditations, sleep stories for adults and children, soothing sounds and more.

Farmers' Almanac: 16 Full Moon Rituals to help you Recharge, Reflect, and Reconnect

www.farmersalmanac.com

Well-being Rituals for the New Moon

www.eco-age.com

Teaching Yoga to Children with Autism (YouTube video)

Sep 11, 2015. Yoga can be a great start to build the fitness levels of children with autism. Here, Coach Dave shares Roan's routine. NCHPAD (National Center on Health, Physical Activity and Disability) is the nation's premier center in promoting the health and wellness of people with disabilities. To view more resources and services which can benefit all ages and populations:
Website: http://www.nchpad.org

Email: email@nchpad.org
Phone: 1-800-900-8086
Facebook: https://facebook.com/nchpad
Twitter: https://twitter.com/nchpad
Instagram: https://instagram.com/nchpad/

Enter the "Flow State" High Theta low Alpha wave Binaural beats music (YouTube video)

This music video to use during meditation stimulates brain wave frequencies for increased creativity and cognitive enhancement, focus, memory, sleep, healing, manifesting, happiness, and more.

https://www.youtube.com/watch?v=p3BIW8GbVF8

Autism Hero Project

Promotes autism acceptance, changing public policy, and the way the world does business by being intentional about inclusion.

www.autismheroproject.org

E2M Training Motivation

Positive Mindset Coaching in every workout ~ Behavior Change ~ Motivational Support from home. The E2M8 online fitness program is an 8-week body transformation program that consists of workouts, meal plans, and coaching.

This is a highly effective course that you can use for life beyond the eight weeks (at no extra cost) which will help your self-care and give you energy.

www.e2mfitness.com

Ms. Jamie Geidel, Music Teacher and Mother of an Autistic Child

Private lessons over Zoom in violin, viola, piano, flute, and music appreciation. Extensive experience with autism. Students gain a channel for self-expression through playing and creating music and often unearth hidden talents. They gain focus and discipline and experience calmness, increased self-esteem, socialization, speech development, and satisfaction of accomplishment and enjoyment. Contact for free consultation.

Search "Jamie Geidel" on YouTube.

Email: jamie@geidelmusic.com

Acknowledgments

It is with the deepest appreciation and gratitude to each of these beautiful individuals, who have shown me unconditional love, support, and encouragement, and who have challenged me to magnify my mind, awareness, and clarity of purpose, that I offer these acknowledgments:

Contributors—Tanys Coughlan, Coleen Cuomo, Nicole Dauz, Lisa Drennan, Nicole Hendrick Donovan, Patrice Headd, Cynthia Kahler, Jack Kahler, Heidi Rome, Sherri Scaccia, Richard Schreiber, Elizabeth Joy Shaffer, Adam Szecowka. Each of you brought this book to a higher frequency than I could have ever imagined. You are each magnetic—the light transmitters in our world. You have built your lighthouse within your children's journeys. Now, you transmit your bright light by inviting others to do the same, cultivating the highest frequencies of love in our world. I am beyond grateful for your time, insight, and wisdom in sharing your extraordinary journey that will ignite internal sparks of hope to real help. These individuals are groundbreaking experts and are here to help you. I love you!

Cynthia Kahler, who has been the cornerstone of this concept from the first impulse I had to go on this journey. She never doubted me. I love you!

Jack Kahler, who has had more of an impact on my life than he will ever realize. I am truly honored to have learned from him through engaging conversations that were transparent, vulnerable, meaningful, and brilliant. I love you!

My children, Alexander, Calvin, Dylan, and Jasmine Trask, who each, in their own beautiful, unique way, have been my teachers in this lifetime and have given me the lessons I needed to learn to hold sacred space for them, so they could make their own path. They allowed me to forge ahead with a rekindled spirit of awareness, self-discovery, and forgiveness, allowing me to turn up my light and love them for exactly the perfect individuals they are. I am forever blessed and honored to be their mother. I love you!

My husband, Kevin Laitinen; I could not have done this without him. His support, including tech support, and always making time to help me at a moment's notice will never be forgotten. Thank you, Kevin, for giving me the *time* to accomplish what is important to me. You have given me the greatest gift of all—time to embark on this journey, as it is not only the destination that matters; it is the journey to heal, feel, and grow into this new expansive life of self-love and compassion to give more and do more. I love you!

My forever friends, who have bonded with the creation of *The Highest Frequencies of Love*—Valerie Lauro, Sherri Scaccia, Patti Sullivan, Maryanne Schofield, Maryann Borden, Theresa Venuto, and Alysha Myronuk. Each of you have graciously given me your angelic energetic belief in me. You inspired me by helping turn any fear, doubt, and uncertainty into boldness, courage, and trust to be my true self. Your heartfelt energy breathes in this book. I love you!

Hasmark Publishing Team—you are the best in the field. This team has guided me with honesty as we developed a trustworthy relationship. You truly cared for, and believed in, my vision and message in the creation of this book. I love you all!

Positivity Influencers—Bob Proctor, Deepak Chopra, Gabby Bernstein, Michael Beckwith, Wayne Dyer, Oprah Winfrey, and Michael Singer to name a few.

My mom, Marie Udas, and my dad, Edward Udas, may he rest in peace. Through the good, the bad, and the ugly—you always stood by me. It has been your unconditional love and support that has helped me become the resilient woman I am! No matter how many times I fell down, I never said this is not for me. Instead, I kept moving forward because it is something you instilled in me from childhood. I am beyond grateful. I love you!

I am truly blessed to have you all be part of my life journey of growth, expansion, and self-realization, so that I could radiate my love and compassion for myself and serve others!

About the Author

My name is Donna Laitinen. I help individuals who are ready to make a shift, and who want to reinvent, declare, and claim the life path their heart truly desires.

I am fortunate in that I have a natural gift for rallying and inspiring people to ignite the spark of internal motivation through forward-vision thinking. My approach is based on behavioral change and spiritual energy connections, in which I help people to heal, recognize their internal gifts, and be inspired to take action.

I am the founder and owner of Evoke Change Center and a professional behavioral change specialist, speaker, facilitator, visionary, and positivity influencer. I am certified as a behavior change specialist through the International Coaches Federation and have an associate degree in Exercise Science. I am also a personal fitness trainer and coach (American Council on Exercise), Meditation, Relaxation, Stress Reduction certified coach, ACE Yoga certified, Breathing Lotus Living Arts certified, Livestrong certified, Cancer AdaptX certified, and Reiki certified.

I am so happy and grateful now that I rise and thrive for my day to unfold, looking for the little surprises that life offers me every day! Not always the surprises I want but knowing that I have a purpose and I am equipped to move in a flow with forward vision thinking. I am dedicated to building a wiser and kinder world by making transformational education widely available. I want everyone to have access to transformation tools such as modern mindfulness, emotional awareness, and self-compassion regardless of financial, social, or physical challenges. I have created and continue to create energy healing systems, allowing for self-discovery, awareness, and consciousness to reconnect to one's inner being and higher power. My focus right now is with parents of children on the autism spectrum.

I have spent several years and hundreds of hours studying, observing, interacting, and speaking with professionals, such as the *Sharing in the Extraordinary Journey* contributors in this book. The autism community members I have consulted with feel this work is useful and essential to humanity, closing a gap of separation, and bridging the connection to inclusion and oneness. I have attended seminars, workshops, and conferences in all backgrounds. I have also participated in podcasts, interviews, and broadcasts on autism awareness.

Only the heart knows how to find what is precious.

~ Fyodor Dostoevsky

I believe the world is shifting. So many are tired of going through the motions, feeling stuck, and struggling with the same unfulfilling results. I see more and more people striving to take responsibility for their energy, behavior, and actions. I recognize "Oneness" as we all want the same thing. We want to restore happiness and peace within and aspire to harmony among all of us. It all begins with the decision to make a mindset change.

Contributors

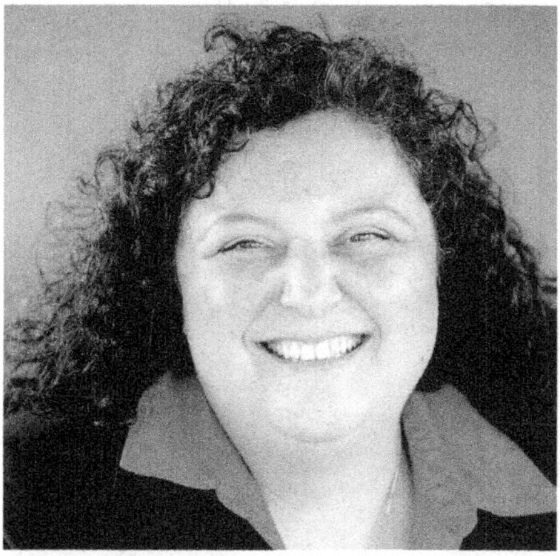

Tanys Coughlan

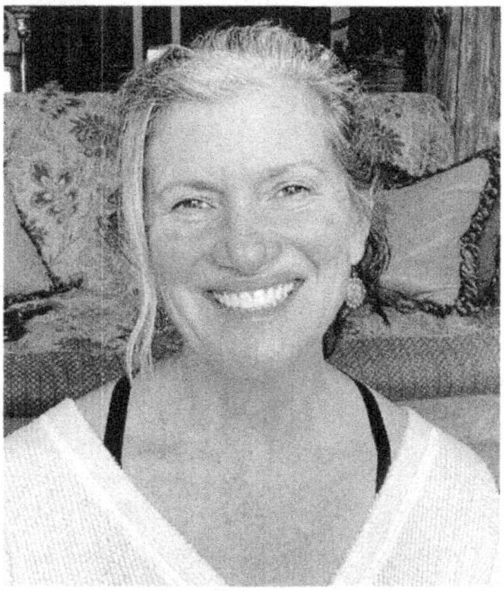

Coleen Cuomo

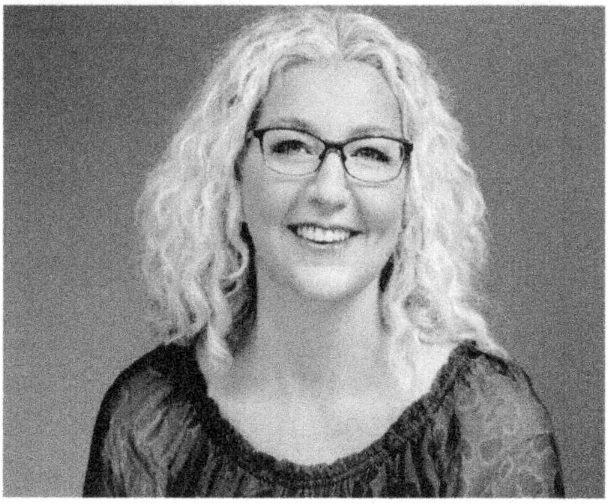

Nicole Dauz

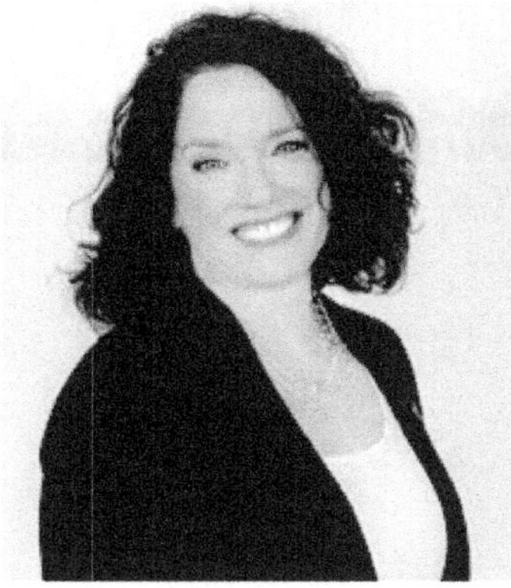

Lisa Drennan

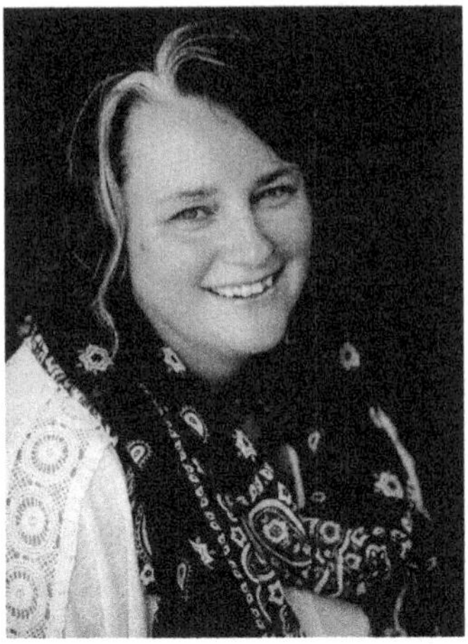

Nicole Hendrick Donovan

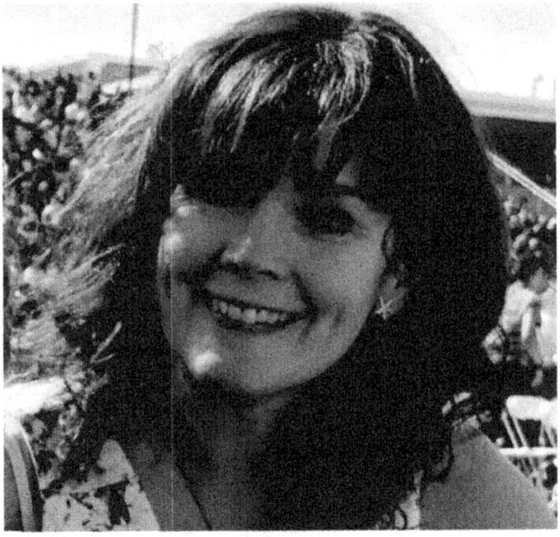

Patrice Headd

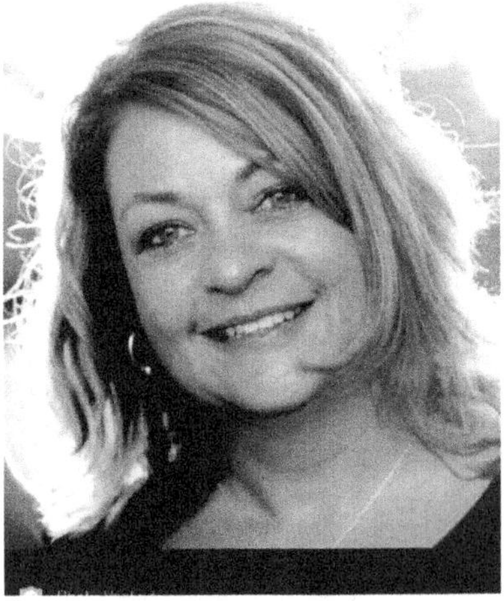

Cynthia Kahler

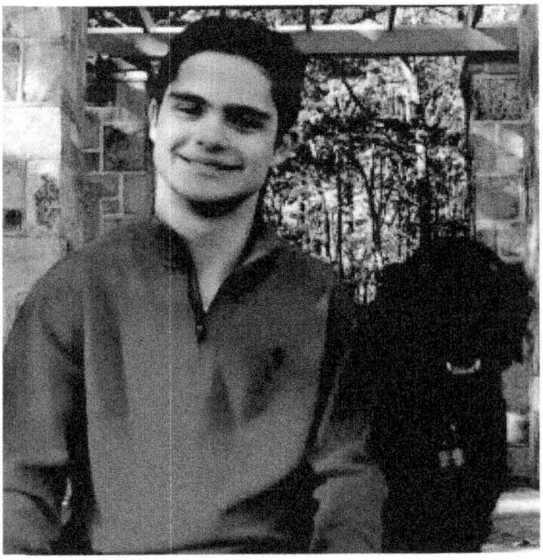

Jack Kahler

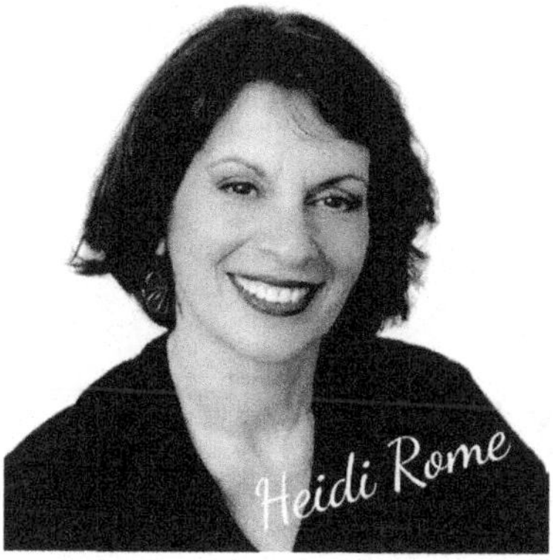

Heidi Rome

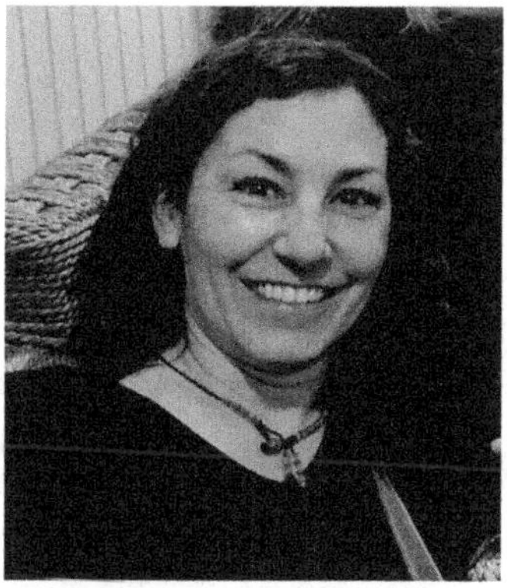

Sherri Scaccia

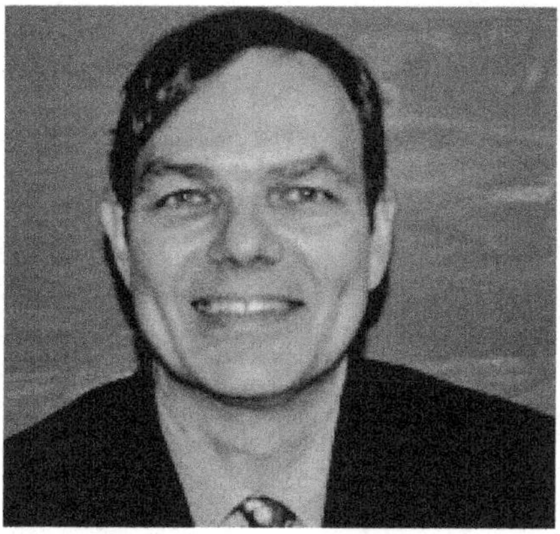

Richard Schreiber

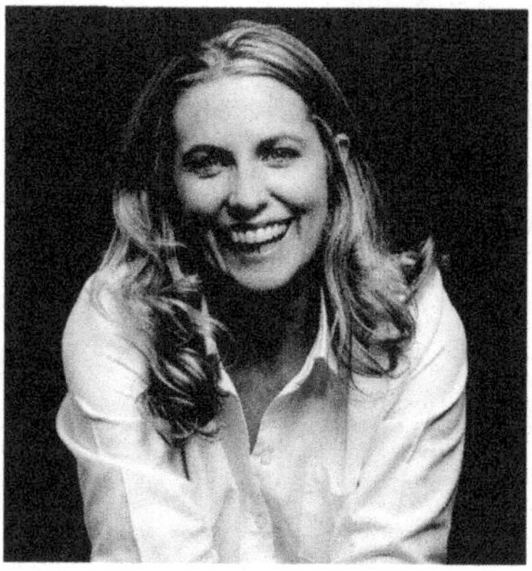

Elizabeth Joy Shaffer

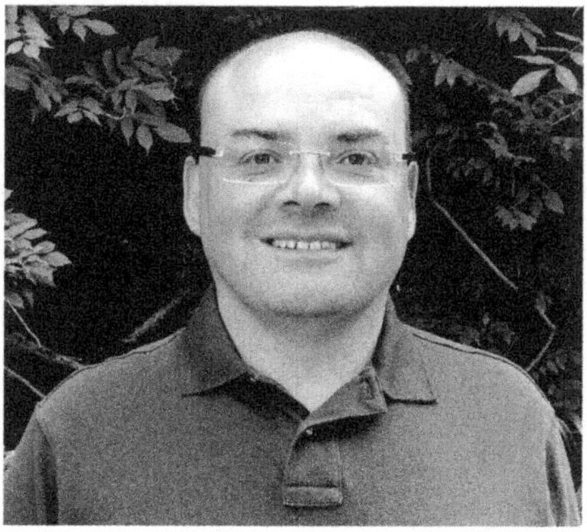

Adam Szecowka

Connect with Donna

To book Donna to speak at an event

Call 781-831-8791

For more information on discounts for bulk orders, conferences, seminars and workshops please go to www.evokechangecenter.com

Made in United States
North Haven, CT
25 August 2022

23204484R10104